Eat Your Way
through the
Menopause

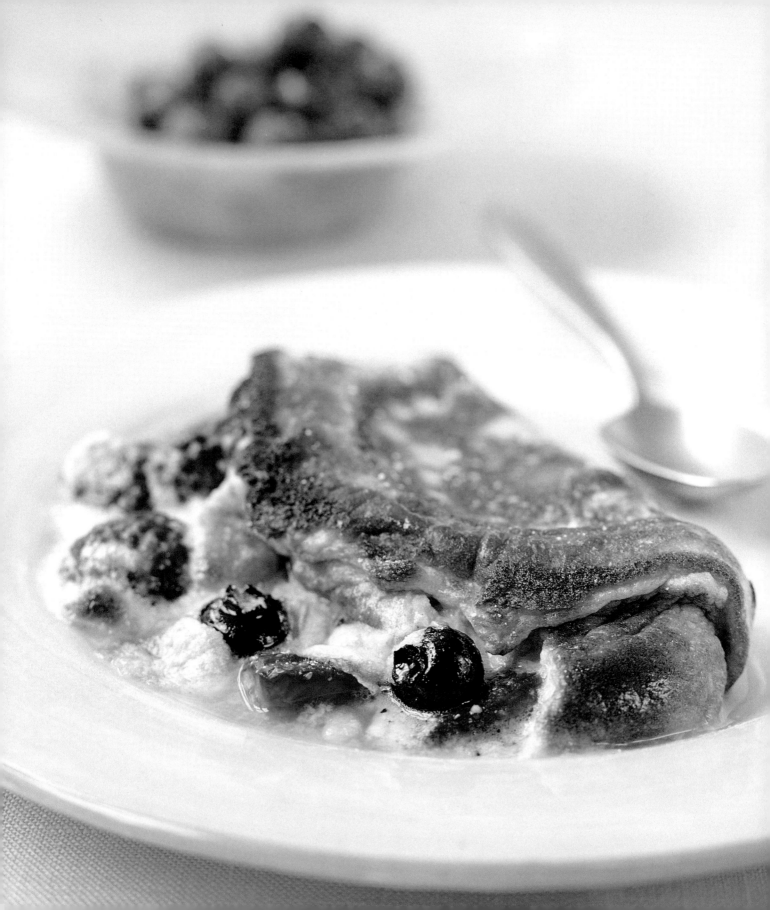

Eat Your Way
through the
Menopause

Marilyn Glenville, Ph.D

with Lewis Esson

KYLE CATHIE LIMITED

To Mum, Dad and sister Janet for all those happy memories

First published in Great Britain in 2002 by
Kyle Cathie Limited, 122 Arlington Road
London NW1 7HP
general.enquiries@kyle-cathie.com
www.kylecathie.com

Originally published in 2000 as
Natural Alternatives to HRT Cookbook

10 9 8 7 6 5 4 3

Reprinted 2004

ISBN 1 85626 468 8

Recipes by Lewis Esson
Designed by Kit Johnson
Home economy by Louise Pickford
Styling by Helen Trent
Edited by Candida Hall
Production by Lorraine Baird and Sha Huxtable

Marilyn Glenville is hereby identified as the author of this
work in accordance with section 77 of the Copyright,
Designs and Patents Act 1988

A Cataloguing in Publication record for this title is available
from the British Library

Printed and bound in Singapore by Tien Wah Press

Contents

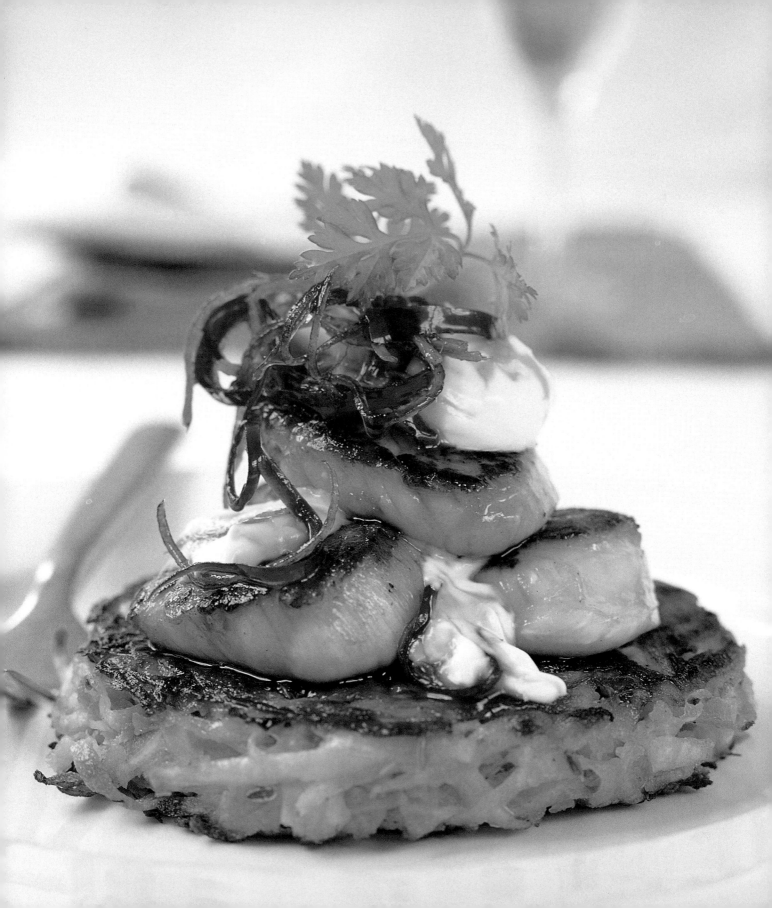

Introduction

Yes, you can literally eat your way through the menopause. In research into other cultures, scientists have found that the menopause is not experienced in the same way by all women. The Japanese do not actually have a word for 'hot flushes', indicating that they do not experience them as Western women do. They also tend to have a later menopause, around the age of 55 on average. Therefore the question arises as to what most differentiates these women from us in the Western world. The answer is our diet. Japanese women also have one sixth the rate of breast cancer that we have. Studies in the USA have shown that when Japanese women move to the West and adopt a Western diet, they develop a breast cancer rate similar to ours. So it is not a genetic factor particular to Japanese women but something in their diet that distinguishes them.

More noticeably, it is people's attitudes towards the menopause that vary enormously according to country. In some cultures it is seen as a positive change: freedom from the need for contraception, freedom from the monthly bleed and the arrival of a new status of 'wise woman'. Yet in our society it is usually seen as a time of loss, a kind of deficiency disease in that when we get to a certain age our hormones decline.

Logic dictates that if we add back these hormones we have a 'cure' – surely? After all, diabetes is the result of a hormone deficiency – when the hormone insulin is not sufficient to maintain normal blood sugar levels – and all that is needed is for insulin to be supplied from outside and the imbalance is corrected. Thus it is suggested that the menopause and diabetes are similar. But diabetes is an illness, the menopause is not. All women are going to go through the menopause, but we are not all going to get diabetes.

Unfortunately, although the menopause is a natural event, there is a lot of pressure on women to take Hormone Replacement Therapy (HRT). This is usually done with an aspect of fear, with the implication that if we don't take HRT our bones will crumble, our skin will sag, our hair will become dry, we'll age more quickly, lose our sex drive and suffer from vaginal dryness. It is hard for any woman to resist that kind of pressure because none of us wants to end up as a shrivelled old crone, which seems to be the message if we don't take HRT.

In fact, research undertaken in 1997 on 160,000 women confirmed that taking HRT for 11 years brings a 35 percent chance of developing breast cancer. [1] For many women, this risk is not acceptable. Also, some women have come to me complaining of side effects of HRT such as weight gain (sometimes up to 13kg/2 stone) and an increase in bra size by up to two cups, with their breasts feeling very uncomfortable. They say that they feel bloated and 'puffy'.

Women want and have demanded another way of dealing with the menopause, one which does not carry these unacceptable risks and side effects and yet prevents osteoporosis and alleviates menopausal symptoms. These can include hot flushes, night sweats, vaginal dryness, mood swings, lack of libido, joint pains, ageing skin and lacklustre hair. Quite simply, the correct diet can not only help to reduce these symptoms and prevent osteoporosis but also protect you against heart disease and breast cancer.

At the moment, 4,000 medical articles a year are coming out on the benefits that substances called phytoestrogens can have on your health. These phytoestrogens, or plant hormones, are contained naturally in certain everyday foods which have a huge influence on how women experience the menopause. In our fast-paced, 'convenience food' society we have moved away from these traditional foods and are now paying the price in terms of our health. By using the simple, inspiring recipes in this book you will help alleviate the symptoms of the menopause by increasing your intake of highly beneficial – and delicious – ingredients.

Heart disease is the West's biggest killer, particularly of men. Eating the foods that are described in this book can also decrease LDL cholesterol ('bad' cholesterol) and so reduce the risk of heart disease. Prostate cancer is another serious killer, with four times more men dying from it than women from cancer of the cervix. Worryingly, it is on the increase: each year more men in the UK are diagnosed with it. Yet Japanese men have a lower death rate for prostate cancer than men in the UK. Why? Evidence points to the fact that the Japanese eat good quantities of foods like soya (one of the phytoestrogens) every day.

These phytoestrogens have a balancing effect on hormones in both men and women. In this way, not only do menopausal women benefit from the advice and recipes given in this book, but the men in their lives do too. The book is invaluable for any family that wants to avoid many of today's illnesses and enjoy eating their way to optimum health.

Understanding the role of oestrogen

Oestrogen is the key hormone responsible for the transition from childhood to womanhood. It causes the breasts to develop and produces our characteristic feminine shape. It also causes the lining of the womb (uterus) to thicken each month in anticipation of receiving a fertilised egg.

The average age of the menopause in the UK is 51 but symptoms associated with the menopause such as hot flushes, night sweats, etc can all start well before your periods stop. As you get nearer to the menopause, ovulation (when an egg is released) becomes less likely each month because oestrogen levels are beginning to decline. However, as they will still have a period most women won't know they have not ovulated.

At the actual menopause, when you have your last period, you have literally run out of eggs. You start off with a certain amount of eggs from birth but over the years they are used up and die off.

Contrary to popular opinion, the menopausal ovary is not a dead or dying organ. It continues to produce oestrogen, although in smaller quantities, for at least 12 years after the start of the menopause. (The start is considered to be the moment when hormone production begins to decline.) In addition, the adrenal glands (which sit on top of the kidneys) produce oestrogen, which is used alongside the ovaries' diminishing supply. Body fat is also a manufacturing plant for oestrogen. Fat produces oestrogen all our lives – which is why low- or no-fat diets, so often recommended for slimmers, can be a big mistake for women.

As women, we need oestrogen to protect our bones and heart. Nature is always trying to maintain a balance because there are problems if oestrogen levels are either too low or too high. If we don't have enough our bones and heart are not protected, and if we have too much we risk breast cancer.

Because body fat is a manufacturing plant for oestrogen, if you are overweight your oestrogen levels will be higher than normal. It is fine to become slightly heavier at the menopause since this extra oestrogen from the fat cells balances the oestrogen decline from the ovaries. However, being very overweight brings with it excess oestrogen levels, which can mean increased risks of breast and womb cancer. Both breast and womb cancer are oestrogen-sensitive, meaning that oestrogen can stimulate cancer cells and can actually grow in the presence of this hormone. Oestrogen's role in the body is as a 'builder', helping to build the lining of the womb in the first half of the menstrual cycle. If this 'building' mechanism goes out of control, then increased cell growth could lead to an oestrogen-dependent tumour and sometimes cancer.

Other conditions that are affected by high oestrogen levels include endometriosis (when the lining of the womb grows in places other than just the womb), fibroids (benign tumours in the womb), heavy and/or long periods and fibrocystic breast

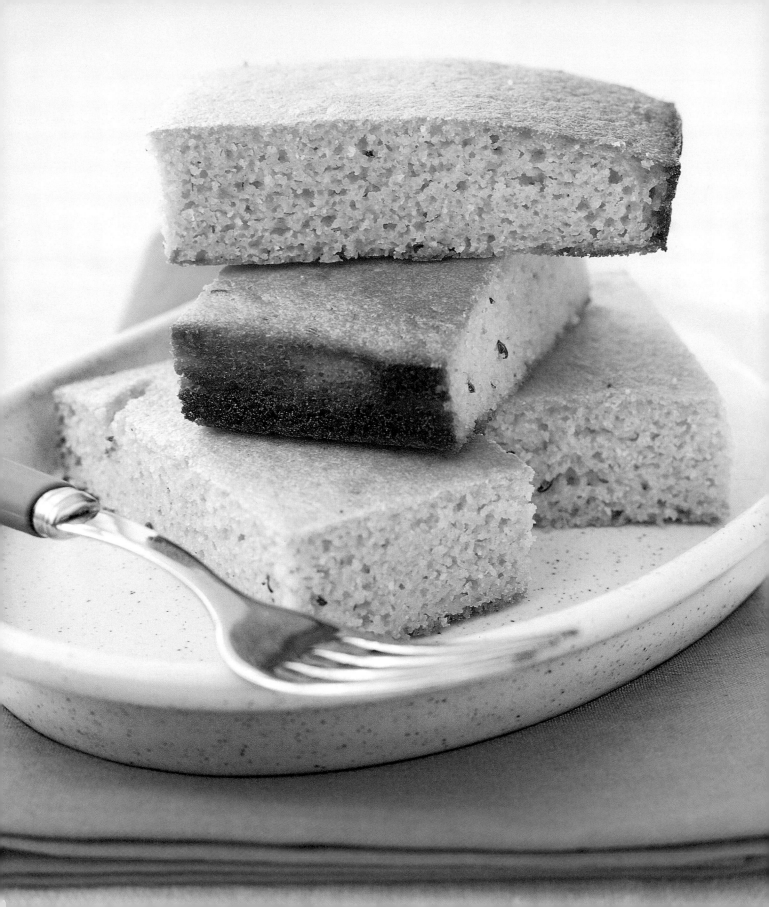

disease (lumpy and tender breasts). Eating healthy foods, such as the recipes in this book, will help to control your weight naturally without having to diet, which doesn't work anyway. If you need extra help with weight loss, my book *Natural Alternatives to Dieting* will be useful.

'GOOD' AND 'BAD' OESTROGENS

There are 'good' and 'bad' oestrogens, in terms of whether they are carcinogenic or not. Oestrogen is not one hormone but several grouped together, including oestradiol, oestrone and oestriol. All three oestrogens have the same beneficial effects on our skin and vagina and protect the heart and bones. The oestrogens vary in strength: oestradiol is 80 times more potent than oestriol and oestrone is 12 times stronger than oestriol. It is the liver's job to convert oestradiol (the more carcinogenic oestrogen) first into oestrone (less carcinogenic) and then into oestriol (which is non-carcinogenic), so it is especially important that your liver is working efficiently as you get older.

Each oestrogen is active at different stages of our reproductive lives. Oestradiol is very active during our adolescent years, but as the menopause approaches production of it declines. Around this time the adrenal glands and oestrogen-producing fat cells are producing oestrone instead.

THE OESTROGEN IN HRT

If you decide to take HRT, you are adding back oestrogen in its most carcinogenic form (oestradiol) precisely at the time when your body is naturally reducing its supply of oestradiol. You are therefore asking a lot of your liver to convert this more carcinogenic oestrogen into harmless oestriol and to excrete it from your system.

Oestrogen therapy has existed since the 1930s when it was given in the form of an injection. By 1938 oestrogen implants were introduced, which were more convenient. However, it soon became clear that supplying oestrogen alone could increase the risk of cancer of the womb and breasts. When research studies demonstrated that this increased risk could be up to seven times higher than normal for womb cancer, there was panic. As mentioned above, oestrogen builds up the lining of the womb ready to receive a fertilised egg, so logically, if oestrogen is added on its own without the womb lining being shed each month, there is a real chance of overproduction of the cells lining the womb and of possible mutation. So in the early 1980s scientists added progestogen (the synthetic version of progesterone) to the hormone therapy in order to protect the womb lining from overstimulation and subsequent cancer. And so ERT ('Estrogen Replacement Therapy') became HRT, as it no longer contained oestrogen only.

There still remains the risk of womb cancer even with combined HRT (oestrogen and progestogen) but it is less than with pure oestrogen therapy. The risks of developing breast cancer from taking HRT are now well known and were confirmed in a study in *The Lancet* in 1997. Researchers looked at the results from 51 studies around the world (the most extensive research on breast cancer and HRT ever) and found that after 11 years on HRT there was a 35 percent chance of developing breast cancer. [1]

Due to the links made between HRT and cancer, research is under way into the possibility of creating a much more targeted drug that would stimulate certain oestrogen receptors but avoid any detrimental effect on the breasts and womb. The drug would function as an oestrogen promoter in organs where oestrogen is needed and beneficial (eg the heart and bones) while acting as an 'anti-oestrogen' in organs where unnecessary oestrogen can be dangerous (eg the breast and womb). This new generation of HRT is called SERMS (Selective Oestrogen Receptor Modulators). The relatively new drug raloxifene is one of these, but its full potential is still being examined. Possible side effects include increased clots and even an increase in hot flushes! So it is unfortunately useless in the treatment of hot flushes or hot sweats; instead it is aimed at those women who want protection for their bones without running the risk of breast cancer. As yet, therefore, we must continue waiting for the ultimate designer drug for the menopause.

LIVING IN A 'SEA OF HORMONES'

We are also exposed to oestrogens from the environment. There are oestrogen-like chemicals from pesticides or plastics called xenoestrogens ('foreign oestrogens') which have been linked to changes in wildlife. Just how potent these xenoestrogens are was discovered by a group of scientists who found that alligators which had hatched in Lake Apopka, Florida had abnormally small penises and altered hormonal levels. They linked the findings with the fact that in 1980 there had been a massive spill of kelthane, a pesticide, into the lake. The xenoestrogens from the pesticide were feminising the alligators.

Xenoestrogens enter the body through food and drink but can also enter our skin from toiletries such as skin creams. These xenoestrogens are stored in body fat, with overweight people tending to have a higher concentration because xenoestrogens are lipophilic – fat-loving. Xenoestrogens can affect men and women differently. Women with higher concentrations of certain organo-chlorine pesticides in their bodies run a greater risk of developing breast cancer than women with lower levels. Girls in the West are now entering puberty earlier than they did in past generations, which may be partly due to the influence of xenoestrogens. At the turn of the century the average age was 15; nowadays some girls as young as eight are growing breasts and pubic hair.

As for men, there are concerns that xenoestrogens are responsible for the decrease in sperm counts by 50 percent in the West over the last ten years. There has also been a rise in testicular and prostate cancer, and even breast cancer. More young boys are now born with undescended testes and other reproductive problems.

How can you reduce levels of xenoestrogens?
The food industry has become reliant on pesticides. There are 3,900 brands of insecticide, herbicide and fungicide which are approved for use in the UK, and some fruit and vegetables are sprayed as many as ten times before they reach the supermarket shelves.

To reduce your own intake of xenoestrogens, where possible, try to buy organic produce. With concern over BSE and genetically modified food (see page 41) there is increasing public demand for organic foods, which is bringing prices down. Organic foods are generally free of genetically modified ingredients, antibiotics and growth hormones and should contain higher amounts of vitamins and minerals – particularly vital micronutrients like zinc as they are grown on more nutrient-rich soil.

You may know of a local farmer who grows vegetables, or there may be local companies which could deliver a box of organic produce to your home every week. Otherwise most supermarkets have an excellent range of organic produce. Waitrose won 'Organic Supermarket of the Year Award' in 1998, the award's first year, and has tasty vegetables and organic breads to choose from. Sainsbury's now has a section of organic packaged foods including organic tomato ketchup, spaghetti sauce, mayonnaise etc. If you are on a tight budget, try at least to buy organic grains such as brown rice, oats etc or organic wholemeal bread. This is because the smaller the food, such as rice or wheat, the more pesticides it can absorb as compared with a carrot for example.

If your vegetables and fruit are not organic, wash them thoroughly. You can buy a wash (like Veggi Wash) from health food shops which claims to be able to remove farm chemicals, waxes and surface grime. Washing cannot alter the amount of pesticides inherently absorbed into the vegetables but it can at least take away surface residues.

It is not only pesticides but also plastics that can mimic oestrogen, so you should try to reduce your exposure to plastics. One scientist in the USA was studying breast cancer cells and stored them in plastic test tubes. Then one day these cancer cells started to divide and multiply of their own accord, just as if oestrogen were present. On analysis of the tubes it was found that they contained nonylphenol, which is one of the family of alkylphenols which are used in paints, toiletries, agricultural chemicals and detergents. As soon as they changed the tubes, the effect stopped.

Try to avoid as much as possible food and drinks in plastic containers or wrapped in plastic, especially fatty foods, because the xenoestrogens are lipophilic. Remove food from plastic packaging as soon as possible. Do not heat food in plastic, particularly in a microwave oven. Store your food in the fridge in a glass dish covered with a glass lid or saucer rather than clingfilm.

WHERE CAN YOU GET BENEFICIAL OESTROGENS FROM?

Naturally, all of us want the beneficial effects of oestrogen – soft skin, strong bones, a healthy heart, etc – without running the risk of developing cancer from taking steroid hormones (which is, after all, what HRT is). Even better, we would like to receive the cancer-protection effects of oestrogen. Marvellously, it is possible to do this, just by eating!

Sounds too simple to be true? Well, it really is simple. The 'good' oestrogens that we require are phytoestrogens, or plant hormones, and they naturally occur in certain foods. By maintaining a healthy diet of phytoestrogen-rich foods, we can mirror what women in traditional cultures such as India and Japan have been doing for centuries and, like them, enjoy strong bones, healthy hearts and minimal menopausal symptoms. The next section explains how this is possible.

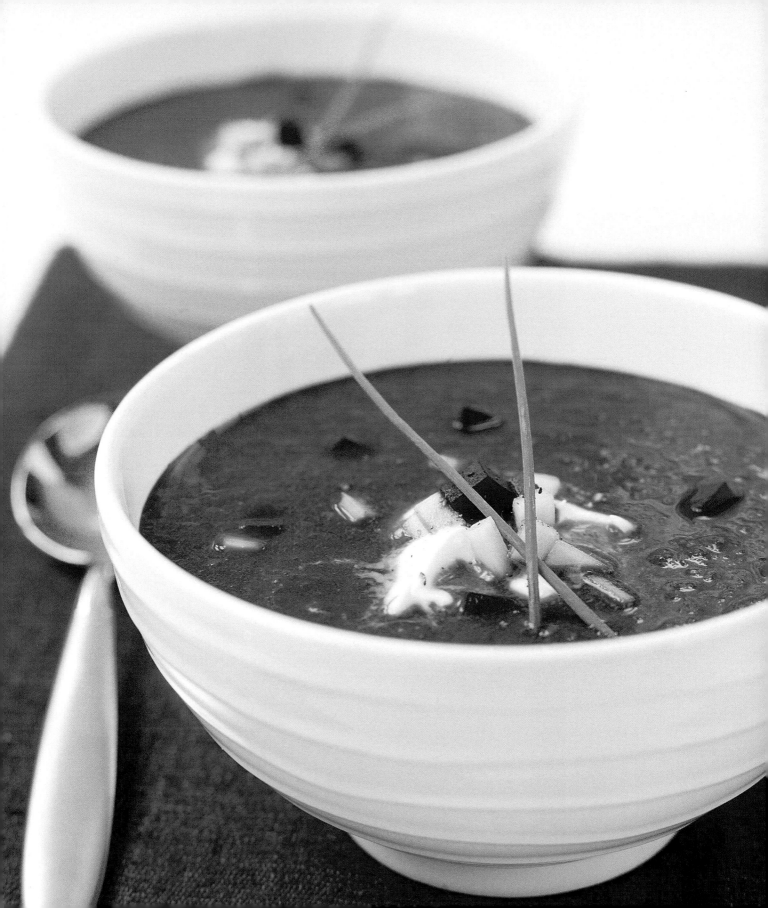

What you need to eat at the menopause

This section covers the foods that you need to eat before and during the menopause in order to achieve specific health benefits. These foods are so easy to incorporate into your daily meals that you will wonder why we are not all eating like this anyway – and that means the whole family. For each group of foods an explanation is given as to their importance at the menopause and the effect they will have on your body.

Many foods are recommended for one particular benefit, yet also contain other valuable qualities. Soya is a good example of this. Not only does it have valuable levels of phytoestrogens but it also contains good levels of essential fatty acids, has antioxidant properties, is virtually saturated fat-free, and has excellent levels of vegetable protein and a good fibre content. There are many other foods like this, but in general I have focused on their principal beneficial qualities.

Follow this book's advice in order to:

◆ control menopausal symptoms like hot flushes, night sweats, vaginal dryness, lack of sex drive, lack of energy, mood swings

◆ prevent osteoporosis

◆ maintain a healthy heart

◆ protect against cancer

◆ minimise aching joints and stiffness

◆ prevent degenerative diseases like arthritis

◆ bring you good mental health

◆ slow down the ageing process

◆ control weight naturally – no need for dieting

◆ aim for optimum health, which in turn will give you a good quality of life so that you have enough energy for your needs, healthy sleep and a zest for living

Can all of this be achieved just by eating certain foods? The answer is yes, and it is all backed up by scientific studies.

PHYTOESTROGENS – PLANT HORMONES

Phytoestrogens ('phyto' meaning plant) are naturally occurring substances in food that have a hormone-like action. Almost all fruit, vegetables and cereals contain phytoestrogens in varying strengths and composition, but it is the isoflavones (one of the classes of phytoestrogens) that are the most beneficial kind. These are found in legumes such as soya, lentils, chickpeas, etc. In the human gut, bacteria convert isoflavones into substances that have an oestrogenic action, although they are not themselves hormones.

An average Japanese woman's daily intake of isoflavones is between 20 and 80 mg per day, Asian women's diets about 45 mg per day, while American and British women generally only consume

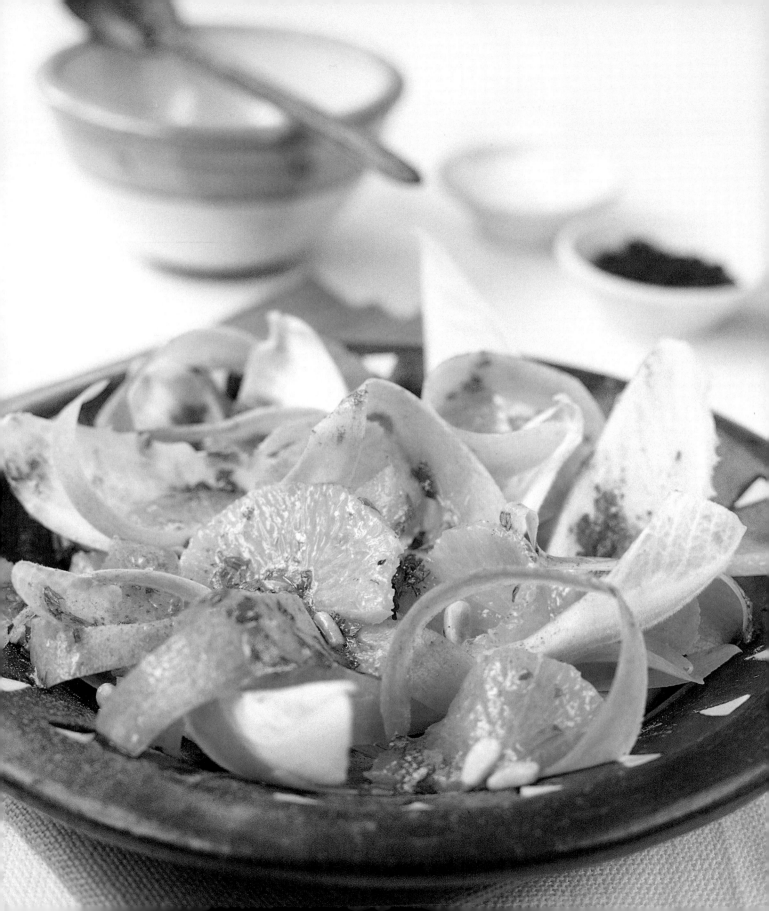

between 1 and 3mg per day – quite a difference.[1] Tests show that Japanese women have as much as 100–1,000 times higher levels of isoflavones in their urine and plasma than the amount found among British and Americans. This indicates that their traditional soya-high diet supplies them naturally with the phytonutrients (plant compounds) that may prevent hormonally linked cancers.[2]

Phytoestrogens can be broken down into a number of classes, including:

Isoflavones   These are found in high concentration in legumes such as lentils, chickpeas and soya beans, which are particularly rich in isoflavones. There are four important types of isoflavones contained in food: genistein, daidzein, biochanin A and formononetin. Chickpeas and lentils contain all four types, while soya contains just genistein and daidzein.

Lignans   These are found in almost all cereals and vegetables, with the highest concentrations in the oilseeds, especially linseeds (flax).

Coumestans   These types of phytoestrogens are found mainly in alfafa and mung bean sprouts.

Foods that contain phytoestrogens
The following foods are sources of phytoestrogens, but tests are still under way to determine their isoflavone content. At the moment it is known that legumes contain good levels of isoflavones, and soya ranks the highest.

◆ Soya

◆ Other legumes such as lentils, chickpeas, aduki beans, kidney beans, peas

◆ Garlic

◆ Celery

◆ Seeds, including linseeds, sesame, pumpkin, poppy, caraway, sunflower

◆ Grains like rice, oats, wheat, barley, rye

◆ Fruit, including apples, plums, cherries, cranberries, citrus fruits

◆ Vegetables, including broccoli, carrots, rhubarb, potatoes

◆ Sprouts like alfafa and mung bean sprouts

◆ Some herbs and spices are also classed as phytoestrogens, including cinnamon, sage, red clover, hops, fennel, parsley

Soya
Soya beans are especially rich in phytoestrogens and so have been studied extensively. Soya contains two isoflavone compounds called genistein and daidzein, which make up approximately 75 percent of the soya bean protein.

Soya beans contain more protein than cows' milk without the saturated fat or cholesterol. They are also the only food considered to be a complete protein because they contain all eight essential amino acids. Soya is also high in essential fatty acids and soya milk is naturally cholesterol-free.

Not all soya is the same   Try to buy soya closest to its natural form. Soya beans are the most natural but they take hours to cook and are not very versatile so you need to go a step down. The next best forms of soya are soya milk, tofu, soya flour, soy sauce and miso (see below).

Soya milk can be used in cooking in the same way as cows' milk, and once mixed in with the other ingredients it is hard to taste the difference. Tofu (soya bean curd) can be used in stir-fries, soups and also desserts. Soya flour can be very useful as it can be added to other flours to make cakes, pastries, etc.

Soy sauce, made from fermented soya beans, is fine as a flavouring but as you only need small amounts at a time it is not possible to obtain enough phytoestrogens.

Miso is also made from fermented soya beans and is used as a paste to add to soups or casseroles.

The more processing that is done to the soya, the fewer phytoestrogens are in the food, as is the case with TVP (textured vegetable protein) which is made up into meat look-a-likes. If alcohol is used in the extraction process, all the plant oestrogen value of the soya can be destroyed.

A high percentage of products containing soya are genetically modified. It is advisable to try to avoid such products where possible: check the label carefully and otherwise buy organic products. (For more details on GM foods, see page 41.)

How much phytoestrogen do you need?
As there are many foods which contain varying amounts of phytoestrogens, it is possible to have interesting and varied meals and still benefit. As a guideline, research has estimated that you should try to include 45mg of isoflavones per day in your diet. A typical serving (55g/2oz) of tofu or soya milk (600ml/1 pint) will contain approximately 35 to 40mg of isoflavones, so you do not need to eat masses of soya in order to achieve a good daily amount. That said, some Oriental cultures can consume as much as 80mg a day in the form of miso soup, tofu, tempeh, etc, with no documented negative effects.

Phytoestrogens and the symptoms of the menopause
There are numerous research papers on the beneficial effects of soya in reducing hot flushes. In one study the addition of only 45g/1¾oz of soya flour a day reduced the number of hot flushes by 40 percent.[3] Another study reported in *Obstetrics and Gynaecology* in 1998 showed that after only two weeks of adding 60g/2½oz of soya protein to the women's diet, they achieved a significant reduction in hot flushes compared to those women who were given a placebo (dummy mixture).[4]

The dramatic effect of phytoestrogens on hormone balance at the menopause was shown in a study reported in the *British Medical Journal*. Women going through the menopause had their normal diet supplemented with soya flour (45g/1¾oz daily), linseeds (25g/1oz daily) and red clover sprouts (15g/½oz daily). This change in diet reduced the amount of FSH (the hormone which rises at the menopause) to pre-menopausal levels – putting the clock back naturally.

Although these phytoestrogen-rich foods made up only 10 percent of their total diet during the experiment, the effect of the phytoestrogens was strong enough to have a rapid and noticeable effect on the cells of the vagina, reducing vaginal dryness and irritation. These changes were detectable in just a few weeks and lasted for two months after the foods had been stopped, demonstrating that the consumption of phytoestrogens is crucial to fending off menopausal symptoms.[5]

Phytoestrogens and fibroids
Fibroids are non-cancerous growths which grow in or on the walls of the womb of some women and are very common as they get older. Many women will be unaware they have fibroids unless the fibroids cause heavy bleeding.

It is thought that fibroids grow due to an excess of oestrogen, so, logically, as the body produces less oestrogen at the menopause they should start to shrink. Our bodies therefore have a natural way of dealing with fibroids, and adding more 'bad' oestrogens in the form of HRT can be detrimental. Try instead using natural methods, such as increasing your daily intake of soya, a source of 'good' oestrogens.

Soya will not only control any excess circulating oestrogen but also its ability to stimulate the production of SHBG (sex hormone-binding globulin, see overleaf), which binds onto oestrogen, will be helpful in controlling the growth of fibroids.

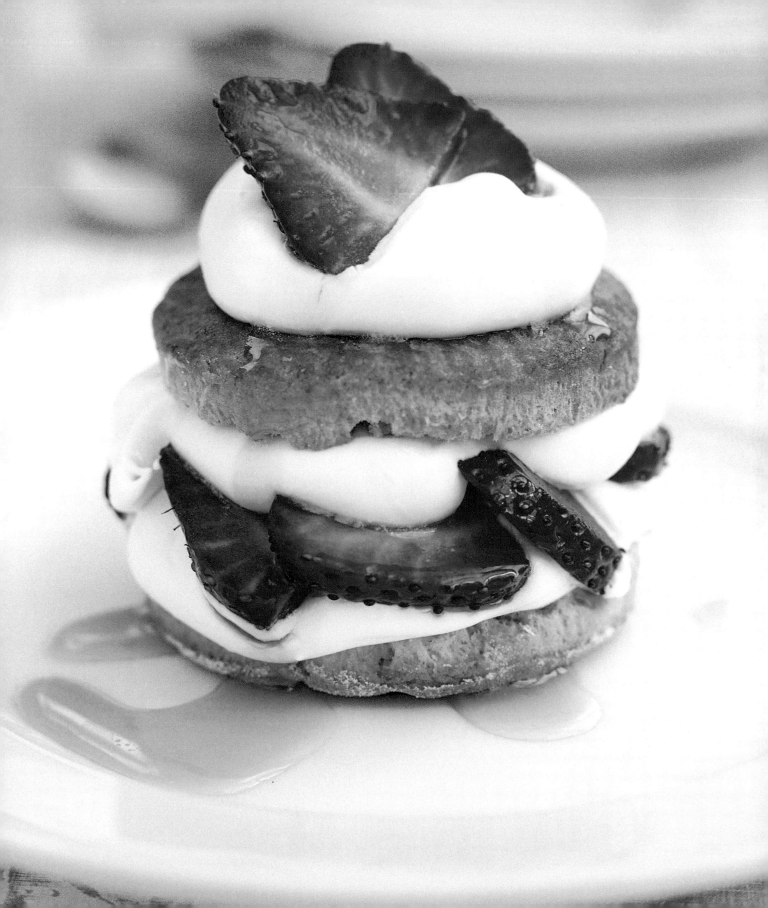

Phytoestrogens and breast cancer

Breast cancer is predominantly oestrogen-dependent. As we get older, our risk of breast cancer increases significantly (see chart below[6]), so anything that is going to lower that risk is to be welcomed. Increasing our intake of phytoestrogens is one method.

Age	Risk of breast cancer
20	1 in 2,500
30	1 in 233
40	1 in 63
50	1 in 41
60	1 in 28
70	1 in 24
80	1 in 16
95	1 in 8

We have oestrogen receptors in the breasts which lock on to circulating oestrogen. Phytoestrogens fit into these oestrogen receptors in the breast and in so doing seem to block entry to the more carcinogenic oestrogens, thus preventing cancer from developing.[7]

Soya beans have been found to contain at least five compounds believed to inhibit cancer. One of these is chemically similar to the drug tamoxifen, which is used to prevent oestrogen-dependent breast cancer. Tamoxifen works in a similar way to phytoestrogens, locking onto the oestrogen receptors and inhibiting cancer growth.

Another effect phytoestrogens have on the hormones is to stimulate the production of sex hormone-binding globulin (SHBG).[8] SHBG is a protein produced by the liver that binds sex hormones such as oestrogen and testosterone in order to control how much of them are circulating in the blood at any one time. The fewer hormones there are circulating, the fewer are available to stimulate breast tissue and possibly cause cancer. This means that the phytoestrogens are able to lower the risk of hormone-related cancers such as breast cancer because they control the amount of free and active oestradiol (the more carcinogenic oestrogen).

Lastly, although we are bombarded by xenoestrogens in the environment (see page 12), studies have shown that genistein, the isoflavone in soya, can inhibit the growth and development of breast cancer cells induced by pesticides.[9]

Phytoestrogens and bones

Bone is in a continuous state of flux. It is constantly broken down and rebuilt through the body's biochemical processes. Bone loss results when the rate of renewal does not equal the rate of breakdown and can result in osteoporosis. Osteoporosis is a condition in which bones are porous – ie filled with tiny holes – and so become brittle, generating the risk of fractures.

HRT is often prescribed in order to protect women against osteoporosis. Unfortunately, many women are led to believe that HRT is the prime preventative measure without being told that osteoporosis could be prevented by other means such as nutrition and exercise without the risk of HRT side effects. And who knows if osteoporosis will happen anyway?

With all the scientific and medical interest in soya, scientists have looked at the effect of soya on bone health. Genistein, one of the soya isoflavones, has been shown to inhibit the osteoclasts (cells which renew old bone by dissolving or reabsorbing it) and stimulate the osteoblasts (cells which replace the old bone with new).[10] In a double-blind trial over two separate 12-week periods bone density in postmenopausal women was increased by taking just 45mg per day of soya isoflavones.[11]

Our bones need calcium in order to remain strong and healthy. Research has shown that the

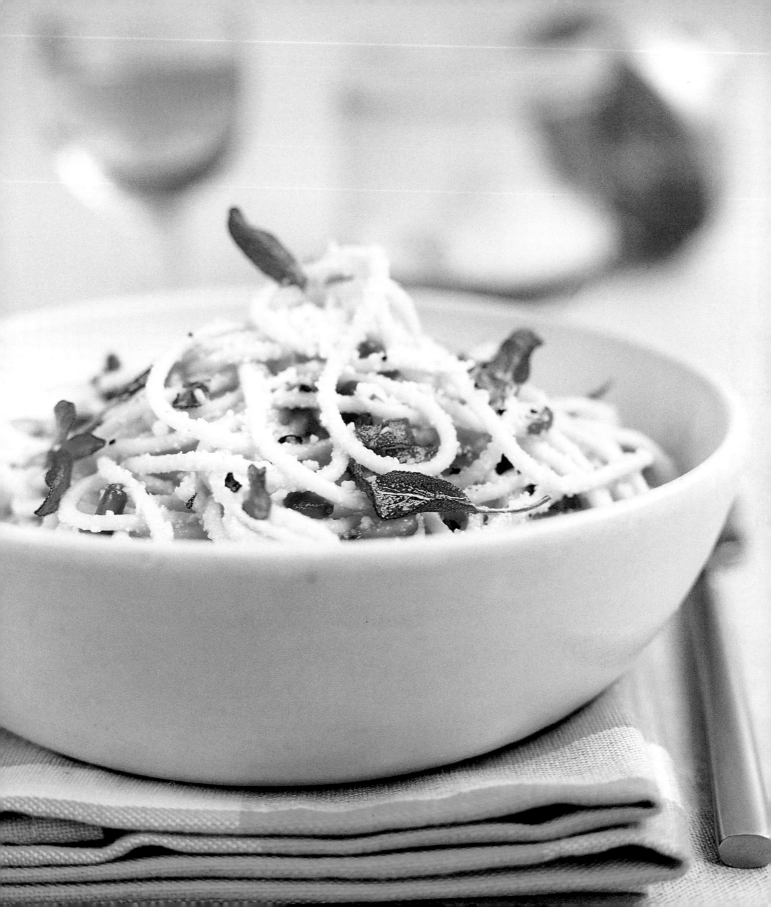

more animal proteins we eat, the more calcium we excrete through our urine and the greater risk of a hip fracture[12] (see Protein Intake, page 35).

	Animal proteins (g per day)	Calcium intake (mg per day)	Hip fractures (100,000 persons)
South Africa	10	196	7
Singapore	25	389	22
Hong Kong	35	356	46
Spain	47	766	42
Great Britain	57	977	118
Denmark	58	960	165
Sweden	59	1104	188
Finland	60	1332	111
USA	72	973	145
New Zealand	78	1217	119

Ironically, the table above[13] also indicates that those countries that have the highest calcium intake also have the highest rate of hip fractures.

Although 98 percent of calcium is contained in our bones, it is not in fact the most important mineral in nutritional terms. Studies have shown that very often women who suffer from osteoporosis are not deficient in calcium, but are in fact deficient in other minerals such as magnesium and zinc.

Animal proteins are found in foods such as eggs, meat, chicken and cheese. Studies have shown that when the same amount of calcium is taken with plant proteins such as soya, rather than animal proteins, the loss of calcium through the urine is lowered by 50 percent. [14]

In this way, isoflavone-rich foods could be helping the bones in two ways: firstly by building up new bone and stopping too many old bone cells

from being destroyed, and secondly by preventing excess urinary excretion of calcium.

Phytoestrogens and the heart
You may have been told that you need to take HRT to protect your heart. The rate of heart attacks in the West is much lower in women than men and by the age of 50 there is half as much risk for women as for men of suffering heart problems. It is not until the age of 75 that they have an equal risk to men. That said, it is still the biggest killer.

With the amount of research into cardiovascular disease nowadays, scientists are clear about the strong link between heart problems and nutrition and have made us aware of how to reduce any risk through our diet by cutting down on saturated fats, etc. But where did the idea come from that HRT could prevent heart problems? It started from a study[15] in the New England Journal of Medicine in 1985, with a follow-up in 1991, which tracked a group of nurses taking HRT over a period of years and compared them with another group not taking HRT. Those taking HRT were found to be less susceptible to heart attacks.

Unfortunately, the study was flawed in two ways: each nurse was fully aware of which group she belonged to, as were the scientists running the trial. In a properly controlled trial the people are split at random with one group being given a placebo (dummy pill). In this way no one knows which pill they are taking. Nor are the scientists told which group has the drug. This is called a double-blind placebo controlled study: both parties are 'blind' until it is over.

In the 1985 study of nurses, the women were assigned a group depending on whether they were already taking HRT or not. It is well known that there are certain contra-indications and cautions against prescribing HRT which include a history of thrombosis (blood clotting), liver disease, breast cancer, high blood pressure, breast cysts, fibroids,

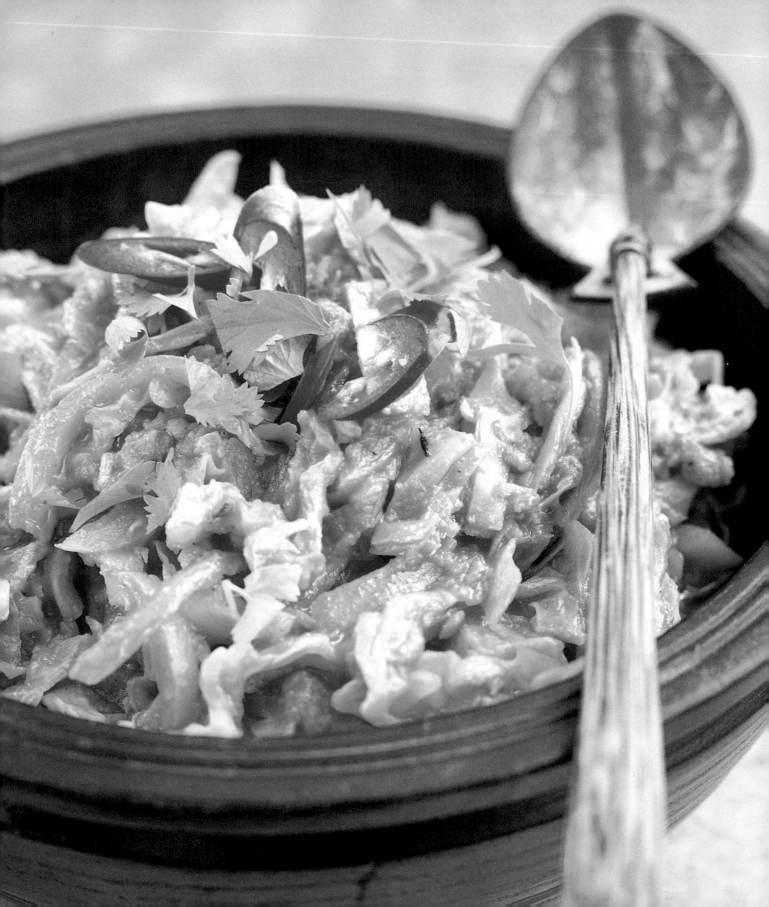

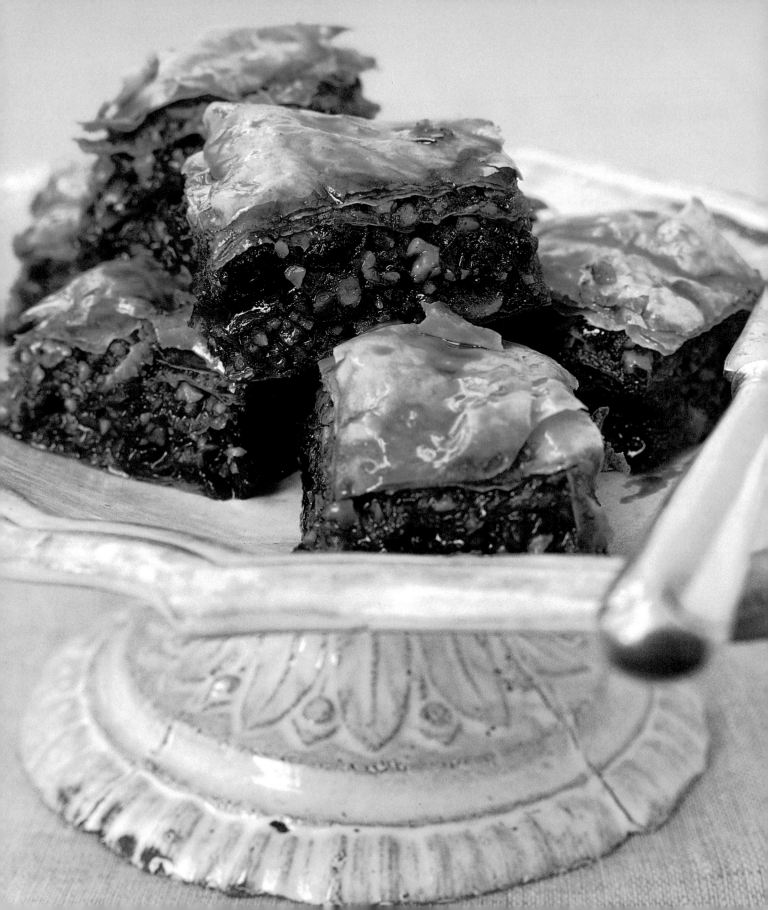

migraine and endometriosis. Therefore none of the nurses with a history of thrombosis and high blood pressure would have been prescribed HRT in the first place and so would have been placed in the 'not on HRT' group along with those nurses who had decided themselves not to take it. For me the jury is still out on this one. Proper double-blind trials on HRT and heart attacks are currently under way but the results will not be known for about eight years.

It is interesting that research has shown that oestrogen does have a beneficial effect on cholesterol and blood vessels, but this effect is lost once progestogen is added to the oestrogen.

Phytoestrogens and cholesterol

Cholesterol is essential for life. It is manufactured in the liver and has a vital part to play in the structure of cells and the composition of certain hormones, particularly the sex hormones – oestrogens, progesterone and testosterone. Cholesterol is carried to the cells by low-density lipoprotein (LDL or 'bad' cholesterol) and carried away to be excreted by high-density lipoprotein (HDL or 'good' cholesterol). It is the balance of these two lipoproteins far more than the total cholesterol level that is so important to your health. If your LDL level is very high compared to your HDL level, cholesterol will be deposited in the artery walls, making them narrower and harder (atherosclerosis) but there is not enough HDL to remove it. The process is similar to the furring up of water pipes and can lead to heart disease.

If you have a medical check-up it is definitely worth asking to have a lipid (fat) profile done which will give you all three measurements: total cholesterol, HDL and LDL plus trigylcerides. After all, it is much better to prevent a problem happening than reacting to it. Remember that a lipid test needs to be done on an empty stomach, so organise the test to be done in the morning with

nothing before you go except water. Ideally, your total cholesterol levels should be below 5.2 mmol per litre, with your LDL below 3.36 and HDL above 0.9. The ratio of your cholesterol to your HDL should not be more than 5 to 1. Once again it is a question of balance.

What is the effect of soya on cholesterol? Research has shown that a high level of cholesterol in the blood can be linked to the amount of saturated fat we eat. Dairy produce and meat are the two main culprits, and if cholesterol is high they should be kept to a minimum.

It is interesting that soya milk is naturally cholesterol-free. It is also rich in unsaturated fatty acids (see page 27). Studies have shown that eating soya decreases the LDL cholesterol and also the triglycerides.[16] It has also been found that the higher the person's initial cholesterol level the greater is the effect of the soya. It is estimated that 25mg of soya protein a day can have this beneficial effect on cholesterol (tofu contains about 15g/½oz of soya protein per 100g/3½oz while two glasses of soya milk provide about 20mg of soya protein).

How exactly the soya protein has this effect on cholesterol is not yet known, but a number of theories have been put forward:

◆ Excretion of bile: it is thought that soya increases faecal excretion of bile acids and in so doing pulls cholesterol from the body.

◆ Fibre effect: soya is a soluble fibre which will bind with some of the cholesterol and fat in the food you eat. As the fibre passes out unabsorbed, this also keeps fat levels under control.

◆ Antioxidant effect: it is now known that LDL becomes atherogenic when it has been oxidised. So antioxidants in our food (see page 30) can reduce narrowing of the arteries. The isoflavones genistein and daidzein which are present in soya both have antioxidant properties.[17]

Can you eat phytoestrogens and be on HRT?
The answer is yes. In fact, it may be a definite advantage to eat phytoestrogens while taking HRT. HRT supplies you with the hormone oestradiol (the more carcinogenic oestrogen), so any measures that you can take to reduce the negative impact of this hormone on the body are valuable. For example, phytoestrogens can act as oestrogen receptor-antagonists in the breast, which may offer you some protection against breast cancer (see page 20).

Can eating phytoestrogens be used to help me come off HRT?
The question I am most asked is, 'Should I just stop the HRT or should I come off it gradually?' You should talk to your doctor about your decision to come off HRT: the most informed doctors will tell you that a gradual weaning process is actually going to be easier on your body. Stopping HRT suddenly is similar to going 'cold turkey' and there have been reports of 'rebound' effects from the quick withdrawal of the hormones. The rebound effects can include tremendous hot flushes and seemingly worsened menopausal symptoms.

I believe that it is better to take three months to wean yourself slowly off HRT. Your doctor can help you do this by either gradually reducing the dose or, if you are using patches, leaving them longer before they are changed. If you still have a monthly bleed it is always important that it continues to happen regularly over the three-month period so that the womb lining is shed each time and doesn't build up. Your doctor will be able to advise you on this.

During that three-month period, you should start to introduce phytoestrogens into your diet. This will mean that when you stop the HRT you are cushioned by plant oestrogens already circulating in your system, and any rebound effects should be minimal.

Phytoestrogens and the men in your life
Having established that phytoestrogens are beneficial for women's health, it is logical to ask how eating more phytoestrogen-rich foods such as legumes and soya will affect men. After all, this means an increase in oestrogen-like hormones in their bodies. In fact, it seems that phytoestrogens have a balancing effect on hormones in both men and women. Excess oestrogen in men can trigger the overproduction of testosterone, and men with prostate cancer have higher levels of testosterone than men without the cancer. A diet full of phytoestrogens like soya can stimulate the production of SHGB (sex hormone-binding globulin) which controls circulating oestrogen and testosterone, and so controls the cancer.

Studies have found that prostate cancer is approximately 30 times higher in Western men than in age-matched men in China and eight times that in Japan. [18] The scientists first thought that it was the Western men's higher intake of animal fats that was causing the cancer, but further research showed that it is the phytoestrogens that are the reason for a lower cancer rate in Oriental men. Japanese men who ate tofu more than five times a week had half the risk of prostate cancer compared with Japanese men who ate tofu less than once a week. Another study showed that when Chinese men were compared against Caucasian men in the UK, isoflavonoid levels in prostatic fluid were seven times higher in the Chinese men. [19]

Phytoestrogens Summary
- Provides oestrogen in plant form
- Controls menopausal symptoms
- Protects against breast and womb cancer, and also prostate cancer
- Helps to maintain a healthy heart and lower cholesterol
- Prevents osteoporosis

ESSENTIAL FATTY ACIDS (EFAS)

It is important to understand that some fats are vital to health, while others are not. We have to learn to distinguish between them, not simply to cut them out of our diet altogether. Most foods will contain varying amounts of saturated, monounsaturated and polyunsaturated fats. It is the predominance of one type of fat over another which makes a difference to your health.

Essential fatty acids are literally essential for your health, and are the next most important group of foods to be included at the menopause after phytoestrogens. Essential fats 'oil' the body by lubricating the joints, skin and vagina as well as performing other functions. Because of the recurring message that fat is 'bad', most of us will have reduced the amount of fat in our diets, to the point where some women are living on completely fat-free diets. However, it is important to differentiate between the types of fats. Without sufficient EFAs, the body will start to send out warnings that there is a deficiency of essential fats. The problem is that these warnings can be quite subtle at first. Signs could include dry skin, lifeless hair, cracked nails, fatigue, depression, dry eyes, lack of motivation, aching joints, difficulty in losing weight, forgetfulness, breast pain – all symptoms which could be 'blamed' on the menopause.

If a deficiency in EFAs is not corrected, the problems can become more serious and can include heart disease, cancer, arthritis and depression. Unfortunately, all too often such illnesses are viewed as part of the degenerative process of getting older – 'just one of those things'.

POLYUNSATURATED FATS

These are the fats that are essential for health. They are found in nuts, seeds, oily fish and some vegetables.

The essential oils in nuts and seeds are from the Omega 6 family of oils which includes evening primrose, starflower and borage oil. The best of these for eating on a regular basis are sesame, walnut, sunflower and soya. These essential fatty acids help prevent blood clots and keep the blood thin. They can also reduce inflammation and pain in the joints and so are vital in preventing arthritis. Interestingly, both sesame and soya are also classed as sources of phytoestrogens (see page 17).

The Omega 3 family of oils is found in oily fish and is also present to some extent in pumpkin seeds, walnuts and dark green vegetables. These oils can help lower blood pressure, reduce the risk of heart disease, soften the skin, increase immune function, increase metabolic rate, improve energy levels and alleviate eczema.

Oily fish include mackerel, tuna, sardines, herrings and salmon. A small portion of salmon (115g/4oz) can contain up to 3,600mg of Omega 3 fatty acids, while the same size piece of cod will contain only 300mg. A small portion of fish can supply us with almost half of our protein requirements for a day as well as providing us with good levels of B12 and iodine, which is essential for the healthy function of the thyroid and metabolism.

Fish oils are also extremely useful in the treatment of psoriasis. A number of clinical trials have shown significant improvements in patients when they were given 10–12g/½oz of EPA (epicosapentaenoic acid) – about the same as eating 150g/5oz of mackerel – in their diet.[20] As these oils act as a kind of lubricant it is clear that they are especially important for us at the menopause, when our skin and vaginal tissues can become drier.

Other studies have shown that eating one portion of oily fish a day can have a dramatic positive effect on rheumatoid arthritis.[21] Polyunsaturated fish oils seem to stop the inflammatory response in the joints and hence alleviate the pain. Many of the women I see complain of aching and stiff joints at the menopause, and I usually recommend that they increase their intake of these oils.

There can be a tendency to gain weight at the menopause, which is often the body's protective mechanism to increase the amount of oestrogen circulating in the bloodstream by producing it from your fat cells. This happens when your ovaries slow down their oestrogen production.

It is excess weight gain that is the problem and this comes about through changes in your metabolism. Essential Omega 3 oils can increase metabolic rate which means that you will burn up more fat and store less fat (for further help with natural weight loss see my book *Natural Alternatives to Dieting*).

A lot of weight problems can simply be due to water retention. Omega 3 oils help your body to produce a hormone-like regulating substance (prostaglandin) which enables your kidneys to eliminate excess water. These prostaglandins also help to lower blood pressure and decrease inflammation in the joints.

Foods Containing EFAs

◆ Nuts (eg almonds, brazils, walnuts)

◆ Seeds (eg sunflower, pumpkin, sesame, linseeds)

◆ Oily fish (eg mackerel, sardines)

MONOUNSATURATED FATS

Unlike polyunsaturated fats, monounsaturated fats are not essential for health, but they do have other health benefits. Olive oil contains mainly monounsaturated and has been found to lower LDL ('bad' cholesterol) and raise HDL ('good' cholesterol), which is one of the factors that contribute to the low rate of heart disease in the Mediterranean.

Olive oil has been used for many years with lemon juice to act as a liver cleanse (see my book *Natural Alternatives to HRT*). Use mainly olive oil for cooking rather than a polyunsaturated oil like sunflower because there is less chance of damaging the oil and creating free radicals (see page 30).

Quality of oils

Quality makes a great difference to the beneficial effects of an oil. Look for cold-pressed unrefined organic oils and extra-virgin organic olive oil. Extra-virgin olive oil is unrefined, and is made traditionally from whole, ripe, undamaged olives. The oil is extracted without heat. Extra-virgin olive oil is generally the only oil you can buy in supermarkets that is not refined. Some supermarkets will also have organic extra-virgin olive oil. Most other supermarket oils such as sunflower are refined in order to obtain the maximum amount of oil from each batch. This destroys the quality of the oil and the nutritional content. Even more worryingly, the refining process – often at temperatures above 150°C/320°F – can increase the risk of cell mutation when consumed.

All oils should be kept in the cold and away from sunlight. Exposing the oil to light or heat – eg leaving the bottle on a windowsill or heating the oil to high temperatures – can cause oxidation. This makes the oil susceptible to attack by free radicals (see page 30). These free radicals have been linked to cancer and premature ageing.

Heating nuts and seeds to high temperatures, by roasting them for example, can also damage the essential oils in them, so it is better to sprinkle them raw onto salads and vegetables. Otherwise make sure that you only toast them very lightly.

LINSEED (FLAX)

These seeds have been given a special mention as they can be highly beneficial at the menopause.

Flax oil is more widely known for oiling cricket bats and making linen (hence the name) and yet it is also classed as a 'miracle' food which we have tended to overlook, and is similar to soya with its range of benefits. The Latin name for linseed is *Linum usitatissimum*, with the second part meaning 'most useful', which you will see it is.

Linseeds are unusual in that they contain not only the Omega 6 oils that other seeds contain but they also contain good quantities of Omega 3 oils. (See page 27 for details on their benefits.)

Linseeds are rich in phytoestrogens, but while soya contains isoflavones, linseeds contain lignans, a different class of phytoestrogen. Lignans are believed to carry the same benefits as isoflavones (see page 17), but are also anti-viral, anti-fungal and anti-bacterial. A good regular intake of lignans has also been associated with lower incidence of cancer of the breast, ovaries, uterus, prostate and colon.[22]

Linseed is by far the best source of lignans: in fact, it is 100 times richer than the next in line, wheat bran. I would not recommend eating wheat bran at all in your diet because it is a refined food (see page 37). If you are troubled by constipation, try linseeds instead of bran. They work like roughage to stimulate the bowel and make motions more comfortable. For constipation, soak a tablespoon of linseeds in water and swallow at breakfast. Otherwise, put some linseeds in a grinder and eat them half cracked sprinkled on food (their nutrients are more easily absorbed if they are broken up).

How much linseed do you need?

One tablespoon of linseeds is estimated to be the equivalent of one portion of soya – ie 55g/2oz tofu or soya flour, or 600ml/1 pint soya milk. You can effectively use them interchangeably. I would suggest that if you have menopausal symptoms you use a combination of different phytoestrogens to obtain the best effect. This will of course also give you more variety.

In a study in the *British Medical Journal*, a group of postmenopausal women were asked to change just 10 percent of their diet to include phytoestrogens. The amount of linseed given per day was about two tablespoons, with soya and red clover making up the rest of the 10 percent. Before the study the women showed signs of oestrogen deficiency, especially in the vagina, with lack of secretions and a feeling of tightness. Within six weeks they reported significant changes: their vaginas became moist and there was a 'plumping up' of the vaginal tissues.

How do you use linseed?

Linseeds are small (just bigger than sesame seeds) so it is easy to mix them with other foods. Linseeds are excellent mixed into yoghurt – either organic plain live yoghurt or soya yoghurt – for extra phytoestrogens. The golden and brown linseeds have the same qualities; the golden ones just look better!

Linseed oil can be used in any recipe where you would use uncooked oil, such as salad dressings, but it is unsuitable for frying. In recipes where you normally might use olive oil only, eg hummus, try combining half linseed oil and half olive oil. Linseed oil is also excellent drizzled on roasted vegetables or jacket potatoes.

The introduction to the recipes suggests a delicious seed mix (see page 46) which will give you both the phytoestrogen benefits and excellent levels of essential fatty acids.

Essential Fats Summary
◆ Maintain a healthy heart
◆ Minimise aching and stiff joints
◆ Prevent degenerative diseases like arthritis
◆ Protect against cancer
◆ Control weight naturally
◆ Bring good mental health
◆ Control menopausal symptoms

ANTIOXIDANTS

Ageing

Few of us welcome the physical changes that come with getting older, but although we can't turn back the clock it is possible to slow it down – naturally.

HRT is often touted as the 'fountain of youth', as Dr Robert Wilson, a New York gynaecologist, wrote in his book famously called *Feminine Forever* (1996). He declared that without this elixir women are 'unstable, oestrogen-starved... a misery to themselves and everyone else, causing, at the extreme, alcoholism, drug addiction, divorce and broken homes'! However, HRT is by no means the only way of releasing us from this 'misery': food is our weapon, particularly when it contains antioxidants (see below).

An experiment which started in 1912 involved live chicken cells being fed certain nutrients every day. The cells accordingly would divide and form new cells, and any excess cells died off regularly. The experiment lasted 34 years and was only stopped when the biologist heading the programme died.[21] It was realised that in this 'ideal' situation these cells could continue indefinitely; in other words, be immortal.

In theory, therefore, if we only put into our systems the right quality and quantity of the fuel that it needs, lived in a sterile environment (no pollutants) and eliminated all waste products, we would never age. Time would pass but the body would always be able to rejuvenate itself.

This, however, is not how we live. It is now thought that each cell is programmed to divide a certain number of times (50) before they start to look 'old', suggesting that we have a genetic clock inside us.

Combating free radicals Oxygen is the basis of all plant and animal life and is vital for our survival. Yet it is also chemically reactive and can therefore be highly dangerous. During normal biochemical reactions oxygen can become unstable, resulting in the 'oxidation' of other molecules, which in turn generates free radicals. Free radicals are also triggered by our environment, made so much more harmful in recent decades by pollution, smoke and UV rays.

It is these free radicals that have been linked to premature ageing, cancer, coronary heart disease as well as to the brown patches on the skin of some elderly people. Free radicals speed up the ageing process by destroying healthy cells and attacking collagen, the 'cement' that holds cells together which is the primary organic constituent of bone, cartilage and connective tissue like skin. They can attack the DNA in the nucleus of a cell, causing cell mutation and cancer. Apart from the normal biochemical processes in the body, other sources of free radicals are fried or barbecued food, radiation, exhaust fumes and smoking.

Fortunately, nature provides us with protection against free radicals in the form of antioxidants. Antioxidants are extremely important because they can disarm free radicals. Our bodies produce some antioxidants naturally, but in the polluted society in which we live we need more antioxidants than our bodies can manufacture, so the best solution is to eat them.

In order to get a good supply of antioxidants you need to eat a wide variety of fruits and vegetables, preferably organic. Try to avoid peeling them as the skin can contain valuable nutrients and antioxidants. This is where the 'French Paradox' comes in. Why do the French have such a low rate of heart disease (only 30 percent of ours) and yet tend to eat more saturated fat than we do? Scientists found that it was wine, especially red wine, that was protecting the French. Unfortunately the benefits have nothing to do with the alcohol but the grapes themselves.

Grapes contain an antioxidant called resveratrol which decreases the 'stickiness' of the blood platelets and keeps blood vessels from narrowing.[22] This resveratrol is mainly contained in the *skin* of grapes, which is why red wine seems to be more effective than white. (Red wine is made from the whole grapes including the skin and pips whereas white wine is only made from the fleshy bit.) So the message here is to forget the glass of red wine and just eat a bunch of grapes – either black or white – skin included.

Luckily, antioxidants are found in many foods that are easy to eat on a regular basis and are included in plentiful supply in this book's recipes. Foods containing the vitamins C, E and beta-carotene (the plant form of vitamin A) all have antioxidant properties, as do the minerals selenium and zinc. Omega 3 oils in oily fish and linseeds can also mop up free radicals. Some important plant chemicals are also powerful antioxidants, such as lycopene (found in tomatoes), bioflavonoids (found in citrus fruits) and proanthocyanidins (found in berries, grapes and green tea).

Sources of Antioxidants

Vitamin A	Orange and yellow fruits and vegetables, eg carrots and pumpkins
Vitamin C	Fruits (particularly citrus), green leafy vegetables such as broccoli, cauliflower, berries, potatoes and sweet potatoes
Vitamin E	Nuts, avocados, seeds, vegetable oils and oily fish
Selenium	Brazil nuts, tuna, cabbage
Zinc	Pumpkin and sunflower seeds, fish, almonds

Beta-carotene (Vitamin A)

Beta-carotene is one of the most important antioxidants we can eat. It is found predominantly in orange and yellow vegetables and fruits such as

sweet potatoes, peaches and papayas. Carrots and pumpkins are excellent sources of beta-carotene: the old wives' tale that carrots enable you to see better in the dark is actually backed up by science (you've never seen a rabbit wearing glasses have you?). Indeed, a deficiency of vitamin A can cause 'night blindness'.

Green vegetables are also rich in beta-carotene, including watercress, kale and broccoli.

Lycopene The carotene lycopene, found primarily in tomatoes but also present in red fruits and red peppers, may have a preventative effect against cancer, heart disease and degenerative eye conditions. However, scientists have discovered that when tomatoes are eaten raw, very little lycopene is absorbed into the bloodstream. It seems that the antioxidant is more readily absorbed when the tomatoes are cooked in oil, such as virgin olive oil.

This helps to explain why the Mediterranean diet is associated with a lower risk of heart disease and certain cancers. Studies show that lycopene in its natural form helps prevent the build-up of the cholesterol LDL (see page 25). In addition, when lycopene was added to cancer cell cultures, the lycopene inhibited their growth.[25]

Vitamin C

Nearly all animals naturally make vitamin C in their bodies except us, guinea pigs, fruit-eating bats, primates, the red-vented bulbul bird and the teleost fish! Most animals will produce around 3,000 to 16,000mg per day, whereas we have to get it all from our diet.

Vitamin C is water-soluble and excreted within two or three hours, so it is important to have adequate amounts regularly. It is valuable in preventing premature ageing and cancer as well as having an extremely important part to play in preventing osteoporosis, like flavonoids (see overleaf).

Vitamin E

This important vitamin is good for the skin and helps to keep the blood from clotting inappropriately – which is especially important at the menopause when one of our biggest risks is heart disease. Vitamin E can also have a direct effect on cholesterol by protecting us from the damage wrought by LDL, the 'bad' cholesterol (see page 25).

Other antioxidants: flavonoids

The vitamins and minerals mentioned above are essential nutrients, necessary to maintain our bodily functions. They are antioxidants as well as many other things; they are involved in so many different processes in the body. There is another group of antioxidants which is often classed as 'semi-essential' nutrients because, although we do not need them to live, they can provide enormous health benefits. This group is called the flavonoids, of which more than 4,000 compounds have been characterised. Two of them are especially important at the menopause; bioflavonoids and proanthocyanidins.

Bioflavonoids   These antioxidants are very closely associated with vitamin C and are found in citrus fruits. They are important in controlling inflammation and allergies[26] and are excellent at strengthening capillaries which can become more fragile as we get older, leading to bruising at the slightest knock.[27] Fragile capillaries can also be a reason for heavy periods: increasing the intake of vitamin C and bioflavonoids has been found to be helpful.[28] Periods can become heavier at the menopause, which may be due to changes in blood vessels but may also be due to fibroids (see page 18).

Bioflavonoids also help to preserve the collagen matrix which can so easily be damaged by free radicals.[29] Collagen is important for the growth and repair of cells, gums, blood vessels and teeth and makes up about 90 percent of bones. It is therefore vital to women eat good amounts of bioflavonoids as they approach the menopause in order to ward off osteoporosis.

Collagen also helps to preserve the elasticity of the skin. The walls of the vagina become thinner and drier at the menopause due to changes in oestrogen. If the walls of the vagina become less elastic they will not be able to stretch comfortably to accommodate an erect penis, so making intercourse painful.

Eating decent quantities of bioflavonoids and vitamin C can help enormously in preserving the collagen inside the vagina – and your sex life. It can also help retain the elasticity in the urinary tract and so prevent leakage or stress incontinence, which is common in menopausal women.

Proanthocyanidins   These flavonoids give the deep colour to many berries such as blackberries, blueberries, raspberries, etc. They are excellent 'free radical scavengers' and, like bioflavonoids, help to preserve the integrity of the capillaries and so lessen varicose veins. With their powerful antioxidant properties, they play a major part in the prevention of heart disease and strokes.

Proanthocyanidins also have a place in preventing osteoporosis because they strengthen the collagen matrix and stop the destruction of collagen. Studies have also shown the benefits of these antioxidants on visual function, which is something that can deteriorate as we reach the menopause.

Antioxidants Summary

◆ Anti-ageing
◆ Protect against cancer
◆ Prevent osteoporosis
◆ Maintain a healthy heart
◆ Protect skin and vaginal tissues
◆ Bring optimum health
◆ Alleviate menopausal symptoms

POTASSIUM

Potassium is vital for the healthy functioning of the heart. A study published in *The Lancet* in September 1999 showed that women with higher blood pressure had a greater and faster loss of bone minerals. The head of the research team from St George's Medical School in London advised such women to eat more potassium, which is present in dandelions as well as in fruits and vegetables such as celery, apricots, dates and figs.

FIBRE

There are two main types of fibre; soluble and insoluble fibre. Insoluble fibre (like cellulose) is found in whole grains and vegetables while soluble fibre is found in fruit, oats and beans.

Fibre is mainly known for its action on the bowel and the beneficial effects for problems like constipation. It binds water and increases the bulk of stools so that they are easier to eliminate from the body. To correct constipation you need to increase your intake of insoluble fibre, which can also help reduce diseases of the colon including colon cancer and diverticulitis.

Fibre also prevents the putrefaction of food which can result if food stays in the bowel too long. Putrefying food will ferment, causing a build-up of gas which leads to bloating and flatulence. Chronic constipation has been linked to breast cancer. This is due to the fact that if toxic waste products and 'old' hormones are not expelled efficiently they can end up stored in the body's fatty tissue, including the breasts. The amount of fibre in your diet determines how much oestrogen you store and how much you excrete and is accordingly very important at the menopause. Soluble fibre, contained in foods like soya, oats and lentils, binds oestrogen so that it is excreted more efficiently.

Our greatest killer is cardiovascular disease (each year 64,000 women in the UK die from a heart attack, compared with 18,000 from breast cancer), and the risk increases as we get older. It is therefore very important that we keep our hearts healthy at the menopause. Soluble fibre binds with some of the cholesterol and fat in the food you eat. As the fibre passes out unabsorbed, it also keeps fat levels under control. Fibre can be useful in weight management in other ways: it aids digestion, increases your feeling of fullness and removes toxins from the body. By making you feel full it helps you to feel more satisfied with what you have eaten and lessens the tendency to overeat.

Lignans, the phytoestrogens, are also a fibre-like substance. Two of the best-known lignans are linseed and wheat bran. To alleviate any bowel problems I advise you use linseeds rather than wheat bran: that way you will enjoy both the benefits from the phytoestrogens as well as the fibre from the same food. Wheat bran should not be eaten except when it is contained naturally in food, eg wholemeal bread. Phytates, substances within the bran, have a binding effect on certain minerals – eg iron, calcium, zinc and magnesium – making them harder to be absorbed. Raw grain contains phytates, so soak muesli before eating to break them down.

Sources of Fibre
- Fresh fruit and vegetables, both cooked and raw
- Whole grains, eg brown rice, wholemeal bread, wholegrain crackers, wholemeal pasta
- Nuts and seeds
- Beans, eg soya, lentils

Fibre Summary
- Prevents cancer
- Maintains a healthy heart
- Controls weight naturally
- Prevents constipation and flatulence
- Controls oestrogen levels

SPECIAL FOODS

Three other groups of foods need a mention because they contain specific substances which can be very helpful at the menopause.

Cruciferous vegetables

As children, most of us have probably been told to 'eat our greens' and there are definite reasons why we should, especially at the menopause. As we get older our risk of developing breast cancer increases. Cruciferous vegetables like cabbage, broccoli and Brussels sprouts help guard against oestrogen-dependent cancers. They contain the compound indol-3-carbinol which changes the way oestrogen is metabolised in the body by speeding up its elimination, making it less dangerous.

Cauliflowers also contain sulphurous compounds that may help to protect against colon cancer. We tend to think of fruit in connection with vitamin C, but cauliflowers can in fact contain more than the recommended daily intake of vitamin C in one helping than in an orange.

Cabbages are also a good source of vitamins C, E, and K. Both vitamins C and E are antioxidants (see page 31) and so are excellent as anti-cancer and anti-ageing agents. Vitamin K is manufactured from bacteria in our intestines and is vital for normal blood clotting. It is also essential for proper bone formation. It is needed to synthesise osteocalcin, a unique protein found in large amounts in bone. Blood levels of vitamin K have been found to be up to 35 percent lower in people with osteoporosis.[30] Cabbage is one of the richest sources of vitamin K but other leafy vegetables like broccoli and Brussels sprouts also contain good levels.

Broccoli is a wonderful vegetable for the health, with good amounts of vitamin C and beta-carotene – both powerful antioxidants helpful for anti-ageing and cancer protection. The darker the florets, the more of these two nutrients the vegetable contains.

The *allium* family

The *allium* family includes garlic, onions, leeks and spring onions. A study reported in the scientific journal *Nature* in September 1999 showed that onions, amongst a few other vegetables, could prevent osteoporosis. The scientists were unsure which exact elements in the onions make the difference, but rats fed on onions over a period of four weeks developed thicker and stronger bones. The experiment clearly needs to be repeated on humans before any real conclusions are made.

Garlic, one of the other vegetables from the study found to be beneficial, also contains cancer-inhibiting properties. Garlic's sulphur compounds increase the activity of macrophages and T-lymphocytes, two components of the immune system that destroy tumour cells. Around 1500BC the Egyptians documented the use of garlic for headache and throat problems, and garlic is also mentioned in the literature of the ancient Greeks and Romans. Garlic has also been found to increase HDL ('good' cholesterol) levels, so lowering blood cholesterol and triglycerides (circulating fat in the body).[31] Although garlic is a wonderful remedy for many health problems, some people hesitate to eat it because of its odour. Remember that you can chew parsley after eating it to freshen your breath.

Seaweeds

Seaweed is low in calories and has a very good mineral content including the trace minerals zinc, manganese, chromium, selenium and cobalt and the macro minerals calcium, magnesium, iron and iodine. Iodine is essential for the healthy functioning of the thyroid gland which regulates metabolism. Unfortunately, the metabolism often becomes sluggish at the menopause, so seaweed is particularly useful at this time. Scientific studies have shown that the consumption of seaweed can also have anti-cancer benefits[32] and can reduce cholesterol and improve fat metabolism.[33]

What you don't need to eat or drink at the menopause

We've talked about foods that are beneficial to eat at the menopause. These are simple to include on a daily basis, as you'll see from the recipes that follow. But it is also important to discuss which elements of your diet can actually make the menopause worse and increase your chances of getting osteoporosis or heart problems. Some of the foods and drinks mentioned affect us all while some are peculiar to each woman.

With hot flushes, for example, look for your 'triggers'. Is there something you eat or drink that will suddenly bring on a hot flush? The common triggers are caffeinated drinks such as coffee, red wine, spicy foods and hot drinks (due to the temperature). Recently one patient simply avoided alcohol for a week and completely eliminated her hot flushes. It is not usual for hot flushes to disappear totally by cutting out one item, but it worked for her. She then had the hard task of weighing up whether she preferred the hot flushes or the red wine!

I would encourage experimenting and maybe keeping a small diary to note when the hot flushes occur to ascertain if they are connected with anything you have just eaten or drunk. Effects can become evident within half an hour of eating or drinking the 'villain'.

It goes without saying that it is no good planning healthy meals, including phytoestrogens and antioxidants in your meals, if you are also eating foods that disrupt your hormone balance, leech calcium from your bones and are detrimental to your general well-being. You will be fighting a losing battle.

This must seem like the bad news section of the book – reducing sugar, tea and coffee, etc. But when you look at the amount of foods that are valuable at the menopause you'll see that in comparison there are only a few that you should reduce or eliminate. If you eat fairly well at home and then go on holiday or are invited out to dinner, the odd 'blip' will not make too much difference. Just make sure that the foundation of your food at home is good.

HIGH PROTEIN INTAKE

We need protein. It is the basic building block for all our cells and bones as well as our hair, skin and nails. It is made from 25 amino acids, eight of which are called 'essential' because we must get them from our diet, while the other 17 can be made in the body. However, an excess of protein can generate problems including kidney stones and Crohn's disease.

Protein causes an acidic reaction in the body and it is calcium's role in the body to act as a neutraliser. When you eat too much protein, your own reserves of calcium from your bones and teeth are called up to correct the imbalance. The calcium is then eliminated from the body through your urine. It is estimated that for every extra 15g/½oz of protein that you eat, 100mg of calcium is lost in your urine.

In 1996 scientists at the Harvard School of Public Health investigated ideal quantities of protein in our diet. They found that women who ate more than 100g/3½oz of animal protein a day had an increased risk of forearm fractures compared with women who ate less than 68g/2¾oz per day. An average portion of bacon is 45g/1¾oz while just two pork sausages weigh approximately 100g/3½oz, which makes you realise quite how easy it is to eat far too much protein.

Notably, the same study found that for those women who ate vegetable rather than animal protein there was no increased risk of fractures. (Tofu, for instance, is classed as a vegetable protein.)

The year after this study the British Government's Department of Health Committee on Medical Aspects of Food and Nutrition Policy (COMA) took the rare step of publishing a report entitled 'Nutritional Aspects of the Development of Cancer', which indicated a possible link between the consumption of red meat (an animal protein) and bowel cancer. It suggested that any intake at or above the current average of around 90g/3¼oz per day should be reduced.

Consumption of red meat can therefore not only increase the risk of osteoporosis but also increase the likelihood of bowel cancer. My recommendation would be to eliminate it altogether, especially in the light of the BSE scare. You'll see from the recipes in this book that you can live quite easily and eat extremely well without red meat in your diet. Instead, you could obtain your animal protein from fish and the occasional egg and dairy products (yoghurt is the healthiest).

It was previously thought that vegetable proteins were 'incomplete' as only the animal proteins contain all the essential amino acids. This has been disproved by the discovery that the combination of a variety of vegetables provides all the amino acids we need. Therefore it is perfectly possible to be a vegetarian and obtain sufficient quantities of protein. A 67kg/10½ stone person needs no more than 40g/1½oz of protein a day.

Sources of Animal Protein
◆ Red meat, poultry, fish, eggs, dairy products, etc

Sources of Vegetable Protein
◆ Cereals, eg wheat, oats, rice
◆ Pulses, eg soya, lentils
◆ Nuts

DAIRY FOODS

Dairy products are constantly the subject of nutritional advice, often conflicting. You have probably been told that you should eat them sparingly because of their high saturated fat content, and yet you need them for their calcium content. However, as they are an animal protein they could make you excrete more calcium than your body takes in.

Dairy products such as cheese, milk and cream should be used in small amounts as they contain the protein casein. Casein is 300 times higher in cows' milk than it is in human milk. Many people believe that our systems were not really designed to cope with cows' milk. Researchers have found that breast-fed babies absorb more calcium from their mother's milk than from cows' milk despite the fact that cows' milk contains four times the amount of calcium.

An added problem is that cows are fed antibiotics to speed up their growth, and hormones to increase their supply of milk. A generation ago an individual cow would produce approximately 9 litres/2 gallons of milk per day; now it yields 56 litres/12 gallons per day. The hormone supplements given to cattle are a definite concern for women at the menopause because of their detrimental oestrogenic effects on the body. For example, breast cancer is often oestrogen-sensitive (see page 20). Because of the increasing tampering with nature, I would advise that you make sure that the dairy products you buy are organic.

At the menopause you are also trying to protect your heart, so it is important to keep the saturated fat content of your diet low (see below). Dairy foods are high in saturated fat, so they should be eaten in moderation.

With low-fat dairy products, the protein content of that food will be higher as part of the fat will have been removed. However, as explained, the higher the protein content the more calcium you will lose and the greater risk to your bones. So although your heart may benefit by eating low-fat products, your bones will not! Ultimately it is much better to buy dairy foods the way that nature intended, eg whole milk rather than skimmed, and to eat them in moderation.

Lastly, you should realise that you are not dependent on dairy foods to obtain calcium. Indeed, many other foods contain more easily absorbable forms of calcium. Sesame seeds are high in calcium, as are some nuts. Almonds, for instance, contain 304mg of calcium in 100g/3½oz. Broccoli is also high in calcium, with 200mg in 100g/3½oz.

SATURATED FATS

You do not need saturated fats, which come from animals and are contained in foods such as meat, eggs, dairy products such as cheese, etc. These are hard fats – fats which are solid at room temperature, and therefore the most saturated.

Saturated fats can be detrimental to your health by increasing the risk of atherosclerosis, where deposits of fatty materials are laid down in the arteries. They can also make it more difficult for your body to get the benefits of the essential fats that you eat. Additionally, saturated fat can be mucus-forming and cause problems with catarrh, runny noses (rhinitis) and skin problems such as eczema.

TRANS FATS

Trans fats (hydrogenated fats) are produced from polyunsaturated oils, as used in margarines. This process involves the hydrogenation of the oil to make it into a solid mass. It is best to avoid hydrogenated fats as they can increase cholesterol and the risk of artherosclerosis, lower HDL (the 'good' cholesterol) and block the body's assimilation of essential fatty acids, making a deficiency more problematic.

REFINED FOODS

Sugar and white flour are refined foods, which means that the fibre and most of the vitamins, minerals and trace elements have been stripped away. Sugar is nothing but 'empty calories'; it contains no nutritional value. Moreover, in order to digest refined foods your body has to use its own vitamins and minerals, so depleting its own stores. Foods containing white flour include cakes, biscuits, breads and pastries. As far as possible it is advisable to avoid such foods.

Sugar

You will notice that none of the recipes here contains sugar. Like protein, sugar causes you to excrete more calcium through your urine because it is acidic. So even if you were following an excellent diet for the menopause, if you included a number of sugary foods you would reduce the benefits of the good foods.

Sugar carries another negative effect at the menopause. When you eat sugar (and foods containing white flour), digestion is fast and glucose enters the body rapidly. Your blood glucose levels rise quickly but are then followed by a sharp drop. This drop is called hypoglycaemia, or low blood sugar, and can make you feel tired, irritable, light-headed and have palpitations. When blood glucose levels fall, your body releases the hormone adrenaline from the adrenal glands and the pancreas produces glucagon. Glucagon helps to bring your blood glucose levels up again.

The problem with this is that the adrenal glands are having to work overtime, releasing adrenaline every time your blood sugar drops. At the menopause it is especially important that your adrenal glands are working at their optimum because it becomes their job to produce a form of oestrogen while your ovaries start to produce less. If your adrenal glands become exhausted they will not be able to provide this protection in the form of extra oestrogen.

Thirdly, it is also well known that it is sugar that makes you fat. This has been explained fully in *Natural Alternatives to Dieting* but essentially what happens is that the more sugar you eat, the more insulin is released. Every time you eat, your body has the choice of either burning that food off as energy or storing it as fat. When insulin is released more of your food is converted into fat and previously stored fat is not broken down.

However much you should avoid sugar, don't substitute with artificial sweeteners. This merely introduces an alien chemical which the body has to deal with. You are trying to keep your body balanced at the menopause, and nobody really knows yet what havoc these chemicals can cause.

Food can taste sweet and yet not contain sugar. In some of the recipes that follow, other forms of sweetener are used in moderation such as maple syrup. You will soon find that as you reduce your usual intake of sugar, you will start to taste the sweetness in foods like carrots and baked parsnips. And if you haven't eaten sugar for a while and then try some, it can taste too sweet and you won't actually like it. Honestly!

Bran

Like sugar, bran is usually sold as a refined food so I would not suggest you include it in your diet. Bran should only be eaten the way nature intended – as a grain in its whole state – or when it is contained naturally within the food, eg wholemeal bread (wheat bran) or porridge oats (oat bran). If you suffer from constipation, try linseeds (see page 29) instead.

SOFT DRINKS

Fizzy soft drinks should be eliminated. They contain high amounts of phosphorus which helps to leech calcium out of your bones. Nowadays it is very easy to consume far too much phosphorus since it is found in most junk foods, including instant soups and puddings as well as fizzy drinks.

Concentrated fruit squashes do not contain phosphorus but are equally bad for the health because of the amount of sugar or artificial sweeteners they contain.

Instead, use pure unsweetened fruit juice and avoid any that say 'fruit drink' on the label as more often than not something else has been added. Liven up fruit juice with sparkling water and for a treat try Appletize, Aqua Libra and Amé. These are natural and make an effective alcohol substitute. Whole Earth also make a delicious 'real' lemonade which is free from sugar, preservatives and artificial colours and flavours.

TEA AND COFFEE

What is wrong with tea and coffee? They both contain caffeine, although tea contains less than coffee. It has been shown that the more caffeine that is drunk the more calcium is lost. Like protein, caffeine causes an acid reaction, so that calcium is taken from your bones to neutralise the acid. Accordingly, drinking more than two cups of coffee (or four cups of tea) a day can increase the risk of hip fractures.[1]

Furthermore, both tea and coffee act as diuretics and so can flush out many vital nutrients and trace elements. There are also substances in caffeinated drinks and foods (eg chocolate) called methylxanthines which have been linked to a benign breast disease called fibrocystic disease. This condition makes the breasts feel very uncomfortable, tender and lumpy in the week or two weeks before a period. As you lead up to the menopause this condition can worsen, making it difficult to sleep, lie on your stomach, or even be hugged. The problem can often be eliminated by cutting out coffee, chocolate, cola drinks, cocoa and tea – a simple solution.

Like sugar, both tea and coffee act as stimulants and so place a strain on the adrenal glands by making them pump out more adrenaline. It is important not to overwork your adrenal glands, especially at the menopause when the glands manufacture oestrogen to compensate for the dwindling production by the ovaries.

Black tea also contains tannin which binds important minerals and prevents their absorption in the digestive tract. So it is counterproductive to eat a good meal full of phytoestrogens and healthy foods and drink a cup of tea at the same time.

Alternatives for tea and coffee

Instead of ordinary black tea try herb teas, fruit teas, Rooibos (caffeine-free South African tea), green tea (in moderation because it contains caffeine) and Japanese twig (bancha) tea.

As well as the best-known herb teas – peppermint (for digestion) and camomile (relaxing) – there are a number of other herb teas which can be extremely helpful at the menopause. Nettle tea contains good amounts of calcium and can also help to strengthen the adrenal glands, which is valuable at the menopause when we need the extra oestrogen from the adrenal glands (see page 9). Nettle tea is also helpful in counteracting hot flushes, as is sage tea.

Green tea (*Camellia sinensis*) is an interesting drink. Both green and 'ordinary' black tea come from the same plant but in green tea the leaves are not fermented. Although green tea contains a small amount of caffeine, it also contains polyphenols which have been credited for the health benefits of the tea. Green tea can help to reduce oestrogen by stopping oestrogen from gaining access to the oestrogen receptors in oestrogen-sensitive tumours.[2] As well as the prevention of breast cancer, polyphenols have been found to lessen the risk of other cancers and also to reduce the risk of heart disease by lowering cholesterol. Both black and green teas contain bioflavonoids (see page 32), but it is preferable to get them from green tea.

As a substitute for coffee try Caro and Caro Extra, Bambu and Yannoh which are grain 'coffees' and contain various combinations of ingredients like barley, rye, chicory and acorns.

Dandelion 'coffee' can also be very useful. Don't buy the instant version as it contains lactose, but buy the roots. Dandelion helps to cleanse the liver – the organ of detoxification which also helps eliminate accumulated 'old' female hormones – and reduce the risk of breast growths. Dandelion is also a natural diuretic, allowing excess fluid to be released without losing vital nutrients at the same time, which usually happens with other diuretics. Dandelion itself contains more vitamins and minerals than any other herb and is one of the best natural sources of potassium, which plays a vital role in the correct functioning of the heart.

What about decaffeinated coffee? Although decaffeinated coffee does not contain caffeine, it still contains theobromine and theophylline, which are stimulants similar to caffeine. In addition, the decaffeinating process is a chemical one, not a natural one. If you experience breast discomfort, the cause could be methylxanthines, contained in decaffeinated coffee.

ALCOHOL

Alcohol, like tea and coffee, also acts as a diuretic. Therefore drinking wine with a meal could lose you some valuable nutrients. The message is again moderation. By all means have a glass of wine socially when you are out, but do not drink every evening with your dinner.

Alcohol is also full of calories: one glass of red or white wine gives 100 calories and a pint of beer around 200 calories. If you want to lose weight, reducing or eliminating your alcohol consumption for a while is a very effective method.

Too high an intake of alcohol will compromise the healthy functioning of the liver. As the liver converts the more carcinogenic oestradiol into oestriol and excretes it out of your body (see page 11), you want your liver to be working as efficiently as possible at the menopause. If you damage your liver 'old' hormones could be circulating since your body cannot get rid of them.

Alcohol can also interfere with your metabolism of essential fatty acids. These are needed to produce prostaglandins, chemicals that help to control moods and vascular reactions like hot flushes.

As already made clear, unfortunately the benefits of wine to the heart are actually due to the skins of the grapes and not the alcohol.

What is best to drink?

Water would have to come top of the list – a simple, natural drink and yet easily forgotten. Your body is made up of approximately 70 percent water and it is involved in every function of the body. It helps transport nutrients and waste products in and out of the cells and it is also used to maintain body temperature – particularly vital at the menopause.

Most of us do not drink enough water. Ironically, women who suffer from water retention tend to restrict their liquid intake thinking that the less they drink, the less their bodies will retain. Actually, the opposite is true. If you restrict fluids, your body tries to compensate by retaining more liquid just in case it is in short supply.

Some women, however, are drinking too much liquid. You can gauge this by the amount of times you need to pass urine. If you get up often during the night or find that you are going very frequently during the day, then experiment by cutting down.

We need to drink around six glasses of water a day, which includes any herb teas you might drink. It does not include ordinary tea and coffee because of their diuretic effect. A wonderful way to start the day is a cup of hot water with a slice of lemon, which is very cleansing for the liver.

To ensure purified water at home, use either a jug filter (available from chemists, supermarkets and health food shops) or have a filter plumbed into your water system, fitted under the sink.

Bottled water The different kinds of bottled water can be confusing, so here is a simple guide:

◆ Spring water – may have been taken from one or more underground sources and have undergone a range of treatments, such as filtration and blending.

◆ Natural mineral water – bottled in its natural underground state and not treated in any way. It has to come from an officially registered source, conform to purity standards and carry details of its source and mineral analysis on the label.

◆ Natural sparkling water – natural water from its underground source with enough natural carbon dioxide to make it bubbly. Again, untreated and utterly natural.

◆ Sparkling (carbonated) water – has had carbon dioxide added during bottling, just as with ordinary fizzy drinks.

The most natural waters, and therefore preferable to drink, are the natural mineral water and the natural sparkling water.

ADDITIVES, PRESERVATIVES AND OTHER CHEMICALS

As well as buying organic food to reduce your intake of oestrogen-mimicking pesticides, try to buy your food in its most natural state. You want to make it as easy as possible for your body to reach optimum health and stay there. Manufacturers often argue that additives, preservatives and flavourings are used in such small quantities that they will not have any adverse effects. However, when you amass all the small amounts in all the different products you eat and drink every day, these small amounts soon add up. We are gradually creating a chemical cocktail inside ourselves, and nobody knows how exactly these chemicals will react together. Your body has to deal with these chemicals, with the result that energy and valuable nutrients are spent when they could be used for more profitable ends, such as disease prevention.

GENETICALLY MODIFIED FOODS

Genes are a set of coded instructions made from DNA which control physical and behavioural characteristics such as hair colour, etc.

Genetic engineering is about manipulating the basic DNA of a plant or animal. This happens naturally in evolution of course, but with nature in charge the process is normally slow and gradual taking hundreds of years. It is this process that ensures the fittest of the species survive. The gene manipulation that humans are now tinkering with bypasses evolution, and as yet we don't know what the price for this will be.

With genetic engineering, genes from other species are introduced into a particular plant to make them more resistant to pests, viruses or weed-killers. For instance, it is now possible to buy a tomato which contains a fish gene to boost its frost resistance. The gene comes from the flounder because it survives well in cold water. This same flounder gene has also been introduced into salmon, and could be on the market in two years' time. In the cold dark days of winter a salmon stops eating and growing, but adding a flounder gene keeps them eating all year round, speeding up their growth rate by 400 percent.

When genes are transferred in the lab, marker genes are transferred along with the DNA. This enables scientists to identify which cells have become modified. Usually a gene for antibiotic resistance is used as a marker. The British Medical Association (BMA) fears that resistance to antibiotics might transfer to animals or humans, leaving patients vulnerable to diseases such as meningitis. For example, genetically modified maize contains a marker gene which passes on a resistance to ampicillin – an important antibiotic used to treat bronchitis, ear infections and urinary tract infections in humans. In another instance, a nut gene was inserted into a soya bean which was potentially fatal for people who are allergic to nuts. In this way it is all too easy for somebody with an allergy problem not to have any idea what they are eating. It is also possible for the DNA from GM foods to be transferred to the natural bacteria in the gut, creating lethal substances and a whole generation of new diseases which could not be killed off by antibiotics.

Some organisations are making a stand against these so-called 'Frankenstein' foods. The BMA has issued a report called the 'Impact of Genetic Modification on Agriculture, Food and Health' and has called for studies to see whether the foods could damage the immune system or cause birth defects.

The Vegetarian Society has announced that from August 1999 all foods bearing the V symbol will have to be free from GM products.

My advice is to avoid genetically modified foods by reading the labels and buying organic where possible. If a food contains soya oil or lecithin, you should be suspicious because there are no obligations for it to be labelled 'genetically modified'. I used to buy my canned tuna in soya oil and have now switched to tuna in spring water. If we as consumers consciously do not buy these foods then eventually there may not be a market for them.

What about genetically modified soya?

This is an important subject because soya is the best-known genetically modified food and up to 60 percent of processed foods contain soya, including bread, biscuits, pizza and baby food. A high percentage of that soya will have been genetically modified. Lecithin, a substance contained in many foods, is also made from soya.

Since September 1998 it has been mandatory in the UK to label products containing genetically modified DNA. This labelling only applies to genetically modified soya and maize (corn) products and only where protein or DNA can be detected in the final product by laboratory screening. Foods containing soya oil, refined starches, additives such as emulsifiers and lecithins will be excluded. Greenpeace estimates that this means 90 percent of foods containing genetically modified products will be unlabelled, so you won't be able to make an informed choice about what you are buying.

Provamel, the market leader of soya products in the UK, has stated that their foods are free from GM products and has implemented a system of tracing the soya from seed to final production. At the moment, if a food is organic, it is much less likely to be genetically modified.

THE POWER OF FOOD

Phytonutrients, or plant compounds, are now the buzz word in science for all those plant compounds in food that can help to prevent disease and keep you healthy. At the moment more than 100 phytonutrients have been identified, including phytoestrogens, bioflavonoids, beta-carotene and lycopene, indoles and proanthocyanidins. We cannot store these wonderful substances so we have to include them in our diet on a regular basis in order to reap their benefits.

Marvellously, nature has packed them into many of the foods we eat. The recipes to follow are full of phytonutrients to help alleviate the symptoms of the menopause and to prevent those problems that can occur around that time, such as heart disease, osteoporosis and breast cancer.

So, I invite you to enjoy eating your way through the menopause.

Bon Appétit!

Introduction to the recipes

Let your food be your medicine and let your medicine be your food HIPPOCRATES

These recipes are specifically designed to benefit women approaching and at the menopause by including certain health-giving ingredients. The introduction to each recipe explains in what ways that particular dish is helpful.

Many of the breakfasts and snacks can provide you with your daily supply of phytoestrogens without having to involve the rest of your family in the diet. It is much more productive, however, to vary your meals so that you access the whole range of important ingredients. I would therefore suggest you use as broad a sweep as possible of the dishes, including starters, main courses and desserts. Most women tend to avoid desserts for fear of putting on weight, but it is the sugar in recipes and the tendency to use a lot of dairy products that makes desserts unhealthy. As this book demonstrates, it is in fact possible to create sweet but healthy desserts without using sugar.

In Japan a typical daily menu for the whole family would be:
Breakfast: miso soup containing seaweed and tofu, rice and often a side dish of fish
Lunch: vegetable and egg dish in miso soup with rice
Dinner: miso soup with rice, a tofu dish with sesame sauce, fish, boiled greens and pickles

This shows quite how many phytoestrogens are conventionally eaten by the Japanese, regardless of gender or age. Japanese menopausal women may be lucky as this is their natural diet, but perhaps you are at more of an advantage, with access to a greater variety of dishes and styles – from French to Italian, Japanese to Thai, Indian and Mexican.

Such cuisine appeals to everyone, and if you can thus subtly introduce ingredients like soya and linseeds into the whole family's diet, the cardiovascular and anti-cancer benefits will be available to them as well as you. For example, cows' milk is not an ideal food because of its high saturated fat content and its potential for generating mucus (and often catarrh), so adding soya milk in certain recipes instead of cows' milk can be a simple change but extremely beneficial.

How to manage when your routine is interrupted

Women often ask me what they should do when they are travelling, staying with friends or socialising and cannot control the foods that are being served to them. The answer is to do the best you can, within the limits.

If you are entertained by friends, enjoy the meal with the generosity with which it has been made. Eating, after all, is a social occasion. Even if you end up with a piece of chocolate cake for dessert, it is difficult to refuse and such a one-off does not matter so long as your foundation at home is good.

If you have to buy a sandwich for a quick lunch at work, buy one with wholemeal bread and with a healthy filling such as tuna. It is much easier when you are at a restaurant, as you can usually have fish with vegetables or a salad. However, only at Indian, Middle Eastern or Japanese restaurants will you eat the most important phytoestrogens such as soya, lentils and chickpeas.

If you are away from home for more than a few days and would like to keep up your intake of phytoestrogens, there are some convenient ways of doing this. For example, a mix of organic herbs called PhytoSoy comes in a handy small dropper bottle and makes a lovely drink by adding one drop to hot or cold water, herb tea or fruit juice. Another easy way is to carry a small box of Novagen Red Clover tablets, which contain all four isoflavones. Just one tablet a day gives you the daily requirement of 40mg of isoflavones. (If you have trouble getting hold of these, please see page 190 for contact details, and they will be sent to you.)

SHOPPING AND COOKING TIPS

To benefit truly from the recipes in this book, here are some guidelines.

Alcohol

Some of the recipes call for a drop or two of alcohol, especially the desserts. This is of course optional, and can be saved for special occasions – they are usually equally delicious without. Some grated orange zest can give much the same effect as an addition of Grand Marnier, for instance.

Aluminium

Aluminium is a toxic metal which interferes with the body's ability to metabolise calcium. It can accumulate in the bones, restricting the formation of new bone – which is essential to prevent osteoporosis. You should therefore avoid using aluminium pans, as the toxins can enter the food through cooking. The same applies to foil and aluminium containers. Instead, use cast iron, enamel, glass and stainless steel. Avoid any coated or non-stick pans, as the coating can eventually wear off into the food.

Beans

Ideally, beans should be cooked from raw but for convenience you can now buy beans already cooked; make sure you buy them in salt rather than sugar. Some supermarkets and health food shops have tins of organic beans.

When cooking beans, add a 2.5-cm/1-in piece of kombu (a Japanese form of kelp) to the pan. The seaweed helps to cook the beans more quickly and also to break down the substances that are responsible for causing flatulence! As seaweed has an extremely good mineral content, the valuable nutrients will transfer to the water in which the beans are cooked. You can either remove the kombu after cooking or, if you are going to blend the beans, you could leave the seaweed in and enjoy all the extra goodness. Never salt beans until halfway through cooking, otherwise the skins toughen.

Citrus fruit

If the recipe calls for the zest of an orange or lemon, try to buy uncoated fruit. Any citrus fruit that is not labelled 'uncoated' will be preserved with a chemical wax, which you do not want to add to your cooking. Uncoated fruit does not keep very long, so be sure to buy it shortly before using.

Custard

All Natural Custard Powder is available from health food shops from a company called Just Wholefoods. It contains cornflour and natural colouring. You can make the custard with soya milk instead of milk, and maple syrup instead of sugar. It is excellent for pouring over apple pies and crumbles made with wholemeal flour. Otherwise, try it over a trifle made using the sugarless sponge recipe (see page 172) and fresh or tinned fruit (in fruit juice, not syrup).

Dairy products

Keep the number of dishes containing dairy foods down to a minimum per day and always buy organic.

Butter Some of the recipes do use butter, but sparingly. Remember that olive oil is always an option instead of butter for cooking purposes.

Cheese Watch out for a rennet called chymosin which is used to harden cheese as it can sometimes be genetically modified. On some cheeses the label specifies that it is GM free. If you prefer, you can omit the cheese from a recipe where applicable.

Cream The cream in any of the recipes – particularly the desserts – is optional and should ideally be kept for special occasions. Organic plain live yoghurt or soya yoghurt makes a healthier substitute, or you can purée silken tofu, as in the Strawberry Shortcake recipe (see page 162).

Yoghurt Buy live organic yoghurt which contains a culture such as *lactobacillus acidophilus*, a natural inhabitant of your gut.

Dried fruits

When buying dried fruits, avoid any that contain the preserving agent sulphur dioxide. Sulphur dioxide occurs naturally but is produced chemically for commercial use. It is suspected of being a factor in genetic mutations and an irritant to the alimentary food canal. The preservative is used most often on dried apricots to keep their pretty orange colour. Those that are free from preservatives will look brown but taste fine. Supermarket dried fruits such as mixed fruit, raisins, sultanas, etc will often have mineral oil added to them. This gives them a shiny appearance and keeps them separate. You should try to steer clear of this kind of oil as it can interfere with your absorption of calcium and phosphorus. Furthermore, as mineral oil passes through your body, it can pick up and excrete the oil-soluble vitamins (A, D, E and K), which your body wants to retain.

Eggs

Egg sizes in the recipes are medium, unless otherwise stated.

Garam masala

Garam masala paste tends to have sugar added to it, whereas powder doesn't. It is advisable to cook the powder gently in a tablespoon of oil for a few minutes before using.

Meat and poultry

We have to watch how much animal protein we eat at the menopause because of the leeching effect on the bones, so neither red meat, game nor poultry are used in the recipes. As mentioned on page 36, red meat takes a long time to digest and can increase the risk of colon cancer. If you do choose to eat animal protein, the best for your general health is fish, with eggs the next in line.

Oils

Look for cold-pressed unrefined organic oils. It is important to store oils out of the light and heat to prevent oxidation, which invites attack by free radicals.

Linseed oil Linseed oil is recommended for salad dressings because of its phytoestrogen content. However, it is very delicate and should never be heated. It can go rancid very quickly and so needs to be kept in the fridge. It is therefore better to buy smaller quantities of linseed oil.

Olive oil It is better to cook with olive oil because there is less danger of creating free radicals, which have been connected to ageing and cancer. The recipes in this book use olive oil unless the oil does not need to be heated. To lessen the possibility of free radical damage further, only fry at low temperatures or, even better, first put a little water in the pan, heat that up and then add in the oil. This stops it from reaching too high a temperature. For salad dressings use extra-virgin olive oil.

Sesame oil The dark version is made from lightly toasted seeds and has a stronger flavour but less goodness. Sesame oil is for dressings only.

Soya oil Unfortunately, soya oil does not contain any isoflavones but it does contain both Omega 3 and Omega 6 oils, which makes it ideal for salad dressings. It is important that you buy organic as it is less likely to be genetically modified.

Walnut oil Walnut oil has a powerful flavour and is good on dressings, but in moderation. Never heat it.

Organic

Buy organic wherever possible, be it bread, flour, fruit, vegetables, soya milk, or free-range eggs.

Sauces

If a recipe calls for tomato ketchup or mayonnaise and you are short of time, look for the excellent organic versions which are available in supermarkets and health food shops. Ideally, use the recipes for them given in *Basics* (see pages 178–179).

Seasonings

Salt and pepper are listed in most recipes, but it is up to you how much you use. I tend to cook with minimal amounts of sea salt and no pepper. I just use salt to cook grains like rice and millet and otherwise use soy sauce and other flavourings such as garlic, ginger and lemon for vegetable dishes. We only need about 4g of salt a day (a level teaspoon of salt weighs 5g), otherwise we retain fluid. As with all things, we don't want too little or too much; an excess of salt can contribute to high blood pressure. Do not add salt at the table but use it only in the cooking, and choose sea salt or low-salt alternatives such as Lo-Salt. They do not contain the chemicals that are added to table salt to make it flow freely.

Seaweeds

There are a number of different varieties of seaweed. Nori is used by the Japanese to make a form of sushi (wrapped around rice with cucumber or fish in the middle). It is usually bought in sheets and toasted in the oven or over a low flame, where it changes from brown to green; otherwise buy the pre-toasted variety. It can be crumbled and used as a condiment added to rice, pasta or soups. Kombu, the Japanese equivalent of kelp, is very helpful in preventing the flatulence which can be induced by beans; its use is described under 'Beans' (see above).

Agar is an easy introduction to seaweeds and is used in some of the dessert recipes. It doesn't look like a seaweed as it comes in the form of white flakes. It can be used to set any liquid, so is excellent to make fruit jellies instead of using gelatine (which is ground-up bones). The rule of thumb is to use 1 tablespoon of agar flakes to set 250ml/9floz of liquid or, if you are using agar powder, 1 teaspoon of powder will set 300ml/½ pint of liquid. Sprinkle the flakes or powder over the liquid and bring to a simmer without stirring. Simmer for approximately 3 minutes, stirring occasionally, until the flakes or powder have dissolved. Then transfer to a dish or mould and leave to set at room temperature.

Seeds

Feel free to sprinkle on extra seeds to vegetables or salads. In order to include beneficial quantities of essential fatty acids as well as phytoestrogens, an effective mix would be one part each of sesame, sunflower, and pumpkin mixed with two parts linseeds. Store the mix in a sealed container in the fridge and lightly grind the quantity you need just before serving. Tahini paste is made from crushed sesame seeds.

When seeds are cooked at high temperatures, it destroys their valuable nutrients and creates free radicals, which is why it is better to eat them raw or very lightly toasted. However, if they are cooked inside breads or cakes, the temperature is low enough to preserve the oil's qualities. When eating linseeds, make sure you drink lots of fluids.

Soya products

When buying soya products like tofu and soya milk, try to buy organic. Some companies like Provamel have guaranteed that their products do not contain any genetically modified ingredients.

Miso Miso is a dark brown soya bean paste. It is made from whole soya beans combined with barley or rice, with a mould culture added. The mixture is left to ferment for one to three years. The paste is excellent as a kind of stock, added to soups or casseroles. Because of the fermentation process, miso contains enzymes which are beneficial for digestion. Once miso is added to soup, the soup should not be boiled again but kept simmering – otherwise the beneficial enzymes could be destroyed. It is best to put miso into a separate bowl with a little hot water or stock and stir to make it into a smooth, slightly runny paste before adding to the casserole or soup.

It is also possible to buy instant miso (soya bean paste) soups. The company Westbrae make two varieties – one with tofu and the other with seaweed – which are available in health food shops. As it is so simple to make (it only needs hot water), I often have a mug of it to start the day when I arrive at the clinic, instead of herbal tea.

Soya milk Soya milk is made from whole soya beans and can be used on its own on cereals and in place of cows' milk in any recipe. Soya milk contains more protein than milk without the saturated fat or cholesterol. The various brands of soya milk will taste different, so do not give up if you do not like the taste of the first one you buy. Some are sweetened with apple juice, and you could experiment by adding spices like cinnamon and nutmeg. I use soya milk to make a milky coffee by heating the milk and adding it to a grain coffee such as Caro or Bambu. For an extra treat I add a drizzle of pure maple syrup.

Soy sauce Soy sauce serves an excellent purpose as a flavouring, but as you only need a dash at a time it is not possible to obtain many phytoestrogens from

it. Make sure you buy one which is free from added monosodium glutamate. The wheat-free version is called tamari.

Tempeh This is another form of soya but has such an acquired taste that it is not used in any of the recipes in the book, but you may like to try it. It is made from fermenting soya beans pressed into a block. Tempeh has a strong taste and can be fried or used in soups.

Tofu Tofu, which is soya bean curd, is made by adding a curdling agent to soya milk. It is a solid white block and can either be bought as firm tofu or silken, which is soft. The firm tofu is easier to cut into cubes and so is ideal for stir-fries. The silken is best used when you want to blend ingredients such as in a dessert, because it is so soft. Tofu has no taste of its own so its flavour is dependent on what you cook with it.

Because of this ability to pick up the flavour of the food it is combined with and because it can be prepared in a variety of ways, it is wonderfully versatile. It can be sliced, cubed, mashed, scrambled, puréed and used in both savoury and sweet dishes. You can buy tofu in supermarkets; many will have organic tofu. If you do not use a whole pack of tofu at once, put the remaining portion in a bowl, cover with water and leave in the fridge.

Sugar

Many products have 'hidden' sugar in them. Avoid ingredients that contain sugar as there are usually excellent alternatives. For instance, Worcestershire sauce normally contains sugar but a company called Life and Health has one with no added sugar or salt. As several of the recipes here include Worcestershire sauce, it is worth getting hold of this version; after all, it will last a long time.

If you crave something sweet, it is possible to make a sweet dessert, pastry, biscuit or cake without adding sugar. Maple syrup, date syrup, rice syrup, barley malt and honey are excellent sweeteners and much better for you. Remember that the key is moderation. Putting lashings of honey on your toast every day is not a good idea, but using it in a cake recipe or drizzling it over porridge is fine. Do not substitute artificial sweeteners or fructose for sugar.

Wholemeal

Use wholemeal/wholegrain products for foods such as flour, pasta, rice and bread. Plain white flour contains the bleaching agent sulphur dioxide, which is produced chemically and may cause genetic mutations. Doppio zero flour is an Italian product used to make fresh pasta, and is increasingly available in supermarkets and delicatessens.

Quantity of phytoestrogens

You should be aiming to eat one serving of soya a day, which is equal to approximately 55 g/2 oz tofu, 600 ml/1 pint soya milk or 55 g/2 oz soya flour. This will give you approximately 35 to 40 mg of isoflavones. Your daily intake should also ideally include 1 tablespoon of linseeds.

As with anything, too much of one thing can be just as bad as too little. For example, if you ate too many carrots you could literally turn orange! So don't just use soya but remember that other legumes also contain good amounts of phytoestrogens. These include chickpeas and lentils – so a portion of hummus added to a salad is excellent for you, especially since the sesame in the hummus also gives you a high quantity of calcium.

NUTRITIONAL VALUE OF EACH RECIPE

There is a system of asterisks to illustrate the nutritional content of the recipes. P stands for phytoestrogens, E for essential fatty acids, and A is antioxidants. An award of five stars (★★★★★) represents the highest value and one (★) the lowest. The phytoestrogen content is only an estimate because plant oestrogens can vary according to brand, eg no two makes of soya milk contain the exact same amount of phytoestrogens. Although research has been extensive into soya products, not all foods have yet been analysed scientifically for their phytoestrogen content – eg rice. Levels of fibre have not been evaluated because it will occur naturally and in good quantities in these dishes.

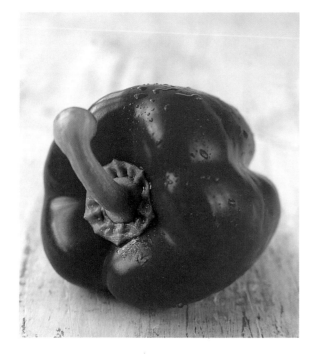

Soups,
starters
and
snacks

No-cook Fresh Tomato Soup

P ★★★   E ★★   A ★★★★

This soup can make a surprising feast of fairly
ordinary tomatoes, providing they are good and
ripe. Tomatoes are an excellent source of the
antioxidant lycopene, which is known to help
protect cells from damage. Phytoestrogens are
present in the soya cream or yoghurt, as well as
a small amount in the parsley and celery salt.

To skin tomatoes fast, put them in a heatproof
bowl and pour over boiling water. Leave for a
minute and then pour off the water. The skins
should then come off quite readily.

The soup has a nice aerated texture as it is,
but for a creamier soup, just stir in 150 ml/¼
pint soya cream or 100 ml/3½ fl oz thick unset
plain yoghurt, ideally soya yoghurt.

SERVES 4
PREPARATION: 10 minutes, plus chilling

*1 kg/2¼ lb very ripe tomatoes, skinned, stalk ends
removed and roughly chopped*

Small handful of flat-leaved parsley

A few sprigs of basil, plus more to garnish (optional)

2 tablespoons tomato paste

Freshly ground sea salt and black pepper

Dash of no-added-sugar Worcestershire sauce

½ teaspoon celery salt

2 teaspoons honey

Put the tomatoes, herbs and tomato paste in a food
processor or blender and blitz to a fluffy purée. Taste
and adjust the seasoning with salt, pepper,
Worcestershire sauce, celery salt and honey.

Chill well (not for more than 3 hours or the fresh
tomato taste will lessen) and stir well before serving.
Scatter with some shredded basil leaves to serve.

No-cook Borscht

P ★★★   E ★★   A ★★★★

This traditional Eastern European soup (see
photograph, page 14) is possibly one of the best
uses of the highly nutritious vegetable, beetroot.
High in antioxidants, unusually a cooked
beetroot contains more nutrients than a raw
one. These nutrients include good levels of
vitamin C and potassium, which helps to control
water retention. Beetroot also contains a
substance called betaine which helps to lower
homocysteine, a natural substance made by the
body. Too high levels of homocysteine have been
linked to heart disease and osteoporosis.

Borscht is packed full of a number of other
health-giving ingredients. The miso broth, garlic
and celery all supply phytoestrogens and the
garlic is renowned for its benefits to the immune
system and lowering cholesterol. Cabbages
belong to the family of cruciferous vegetables
which includes broccoli, Brussels sprouts and
cauliflower. These vegetables help to quicken the
metabolism of oestrogen in the body and help it
be excreted in a harmless form, so guarding
against cancer, especially of the breast and
womb. Cider vinegar helps to increase the
absorption of calcium in your food, which is
extremely useful at a time when you are trying
to maintain good bone density.

SERVES 6–8
PREPARATION: about 15 minutes, plus chilling

*350 g/12 oz large cooked beetroot, peeled and cut
into chunks*

225 g/8 oz red or savoy cabbage, roughly chopped

4 spring onions, quartered

1 garlic clove

2 celery heart stalks, roughly chopped

1 litre/1¾ pints boiling water, miso broth (see page 176) or vegetable stock (see page 177)

150 ml/¼ pint sour cream, plus a little more to serve

1 tablespoon cider vinegar

Freshly ground sea salt and black pepper

Freshly grated nutmeg

Grated cucumber (peel included), to serve

Grated horseradish, to serve (optional)

Put the beetroot, cabbage, spring onions, garlic and celery in a food processor or blender and blitz to a purée. Pour and spoon out into a large bowl or pan and mix in the water, broth or stock, sour cream and cider vinegar. Taste and adjust the seasoning with salt, pepper and nutmeg.

Chill thoroughly before serving. Swirl some more sour cream over the soup in each bowl and scatter with some grated cucumber. Grated horseradish is a nice finishing touch for those who like it hot.

NO-COOK FRESH PEA SOUP

P ★★★★   E ★★   A ★★

This is a lovely recipe containing a great variety of phytoestrogens: from the miso, tofu cream or soya yoghurt, peas and the celery. The celery is especially beneficial as it contains potassium which helps prevent water retention. Celery also has anti-inflammatory properties, so is useful for joint pains and arthritis. The spring onions are beneficial for the bones and the seaweed flakes contain high levels of trace minerals, especially iodine, which regulates metabolism – a boon at the menopause when it can seem 'sluggish'.

Packets of fresh shelled baby peas are now widely available and are a godsend for the busy cook. The real traditionalist can add a teaspoon or two of chopped fresh mint and garnish with mint instead of chives. Save the whipping cream for special occasions.

SERVES 4

PREPARATION: about 15 minutes, plus chilling if serving cold

700 g/1½ lb fresh shelled garden peas (about 2 kg/4½ lb in the pod)

4 spring onions, quartered

2 celery heart stalks, roughly chopped

1.1 litres/2 pints boiling water, miso broth (see page 176) or vegetable stock (see page 177)

1–2 tablespoons arrowroot (optional)

Freshly ground sea salt and black pepper

Dash of no-added-sugar Worcestershire sauce

100 g/3½ oz tofu cream (see page 183), 100 ml/3½ fl oz thick unset plain yoghurt, preferably soya yoghurt, or 150 ml/¼ pint whipping cream

1½ tablespoons mixed seaweed flakes

Small bunch of chives

Put the peas, spring onions and celery in a food processor or blender and blitz to a purée. Pour and spoon out into a large bowl or pan and mix in the water, broth or stock. Depending on the texture of the peas and your taste, you may want to thicken the mixture with some arrowroot. Taste and adjust the seasoning with salt, pepper and a dash of Worcestershire sauce.

If serving cold, chill for as long as you can before serving. To serve, swirl some tofu cream, yoghurt or cream into each bowl and scatter with some seaweed and snipped chives.

If serving warm, add the tofu cream, yoghurt or cream and heat through gently, stirring. Again, scatter over the seaweed and snipped chives just before serving.

GAZPACHO

P ★   E ★★★★   A ★★★★

This lovely summer dish has anti-ageing and cancer-protective qualities from the antioxidant lycopene in the tomatoes, and further antioxidants are supplied by the peppers. Cucumbers contain certain antioxidants which help to prevent oestrogen binding to cells. The spring onions offer bone protection and linseed oil is a source of both essential fatty acids Omega 3 and Omega 6. The oil is excellent for the heart and preventing degenerative illness.

Gazpacho is all the better for being made the day before and chilled overnight, to allow the flavours to develop over time. If possible, it should be served ice-cold. The soup is sometimes served with ice cubes floating in it, but that often dilutes it unacceptably. Instead, particularly if you want to add a sophisticated touch, for a dinner party, say, freeze some of your best extra-virgin olive oil in an ice cube tray – dropping a few whole chervil or flat parsley leaves in each section – and float some of the resulting cubes in the soup.

For an extra boost of phytoestrogens you can use an equal parts mixture of olive oil with linseed or walnut oil in the soup.

SERVES 4
PREPARATION: 20 minutes, plus chilling

450g/1lb vine-ripened or plum tomatoes, skinned (see page 50)
½ cucumber
1 green pepper
1 yellow pepper
4 spring onions
2 garlic cloves
Handful of mixed herbs, ideally including flat-leaved parsley, chives, chervil and basil
2 tablespoons extra-virgin olive oil
1–2 tablespoon(s) cider vinegar
300ml/½ pint canned tomato juice, chilled
Freshly ground sea salt
½ teaspoon paprika, or to taste
2 hard-boiled eggs, shelled and fairly finely chopped, to garnish

FOR THE GARLIC CROUTONS:
2 tablespoons extra-virgin olive oil
1 garlic clove, finely chopped
3 slices wholemeal bread, crusts removed and cubed

Remove the stalk ends from the tomatoes and coarsely chop the tomatoes.

Cut off a quarter of the piece of cucumber and set that aside. Peel the rest and chop it coarsely. Deseed and coarsely chop the peppers. Trim and coarsely chop the spring onions. Then take the unpeeled cucumber and chop it very finely. Do the same with one-quarter of each of the prepared vegetables. Put each into separate small bowls to hand round with the soup and set aside.

Put the coarsely chopped vegetables in a blender with the garlic cloves, the herbs, oil, vinegar and a little of the tomato juice. Blend to a purée. Mix in the rest of the tomato juice and adjust the seasoning with salt and paprika (remember that chilling mutes flavours, so season well). Put the soup to chill in the refrigerator for at least 1 hour, preferably overnight.

While the soup is cooling, make the garlic croûtons: in a frying pan, heat the oil and fry the garlic until aromatic. Add the bread cubes and sauté, tossing to coat them with the oil and garlic and browning them uniformly. Turn out on paper towels to drain.

Serve the chilled soup with the bowls of diced vegetables, chopped egg and croûtons.

MINESTRONE PRIMAVERA

P ★ ★ ★ ★ ★   E ★   A ★ ★ ★

Because of its great number of vegetables, minestrone is an excellent soup for obtaining a good variety of phytoestrogens. The soya in the miso broth is a rich source, as are the cannellini beans and borlotti beans. Other phytoestrogens are found in the celery, carrots, peas, green beans, potatoes and garlic. Courgettes are an excellent source of beta-carotene, vitamin C and folic acid. The cabbage offers effective anti-cancer protection by helping oestrogen to be excreted in its harmless form.

You can also dress the finished soup with a big dollop of pesto sauce (see page 181).

SERVES 6–8
PREPARATION: 20 minutes, plus overnight soaking
COOKING: 2–2½ hours

55 g/2 oz dried cannellini beans
55 g/2 oz borlotti beans
2 tablespoons olive oil
40 g/1½ oz mixed seaweed flakes
1 large onion, chopped
1 garlic clove, chopped
1 bay leaf
3 baby leeks, cut into small bite-sized chunks
175 g/6 oz young carrots, cut into small bite-sized chunks
3–4 celery hearts, cut into small bite-sized chunks
175 g/6 oz young courgettes, diced large
175 g/6 oz fine green beans, cut into small bite-sized lengths
55 g/2 oz shelled peas
1.5 litres/2½ pints boiling water, miso broth (see page 176) or vegetable stock (see page 177)
2 tablespoons red wine
175 g/6 oz young spring cabbage, finely shredded
175 g/6 oz new potatoes, halved
225 g/8 oz tomatoes, skinned (see page 52) and coarsely chopped
Freshly ground sea salt and black pepper
85 g/3 oz soup pasta, such as ditalini or vermicelli
3 tablespoons chopped flat-leaved parsley
Handful of basil
Garlic croûtons (see page 52), to serve
Freshly grated Parmesan cheese, to serve

Cover the beans generously with water and leave to soak overnight. The next day, drain and rinse well.

Heat the oil in a large heavy-based pan and add the seaweed. Sauté gently for a minute or so, then add the onion, garlic clove and the bay leaf, and continue to sauté gently for about 5 minutes. Then add the leeks, carrots and celery and cook for 2–3 minutes more. Drain both soaked beans and add them to the pan. Sauté for about 5 minutes more. Add the courgettes, green beans and peas, and sauté for a further 5 minutes.

Add the water, broth or stock, together with the wine, cabbage, potatoes and tomatoes. Bring to the boil, cover and simmer very gently for about 1¾–2 hours, until the beans are tender.

Season to taste, crumble in the pasta, add the parsley and basil and continue to cook for about 10–15 minutes, until the pasta is tender.

Serve the soup and hand round bowls of the croûtons and the grated Parmesan.

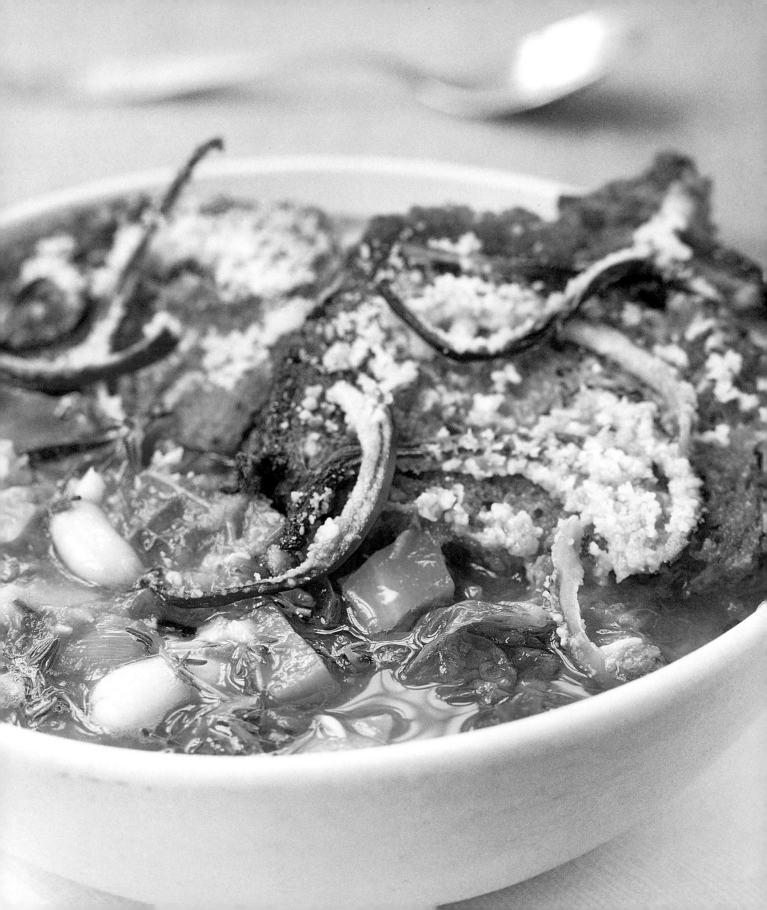

RIBOLLITA

P ★★★★   E ★   A ★★★

Ribollita is a lovely bean soup from Tuscany and makes a good warming lunch on a cold day. The cannellini beans make a delicious combination with the miso broth, celery, carrots, garlic and the wholemeal bread.

The wonderful mix of vegetables and beans gives phytoestrogens in abundance. The carrots, as well as being phytoestrogenic, contain high levels of beta-carotene, the antioxidant so useful in preventing cell damage; the lycopene in the tomatoes has that same function. The cabbage is excellent in cancer protection and the garlic, a member of the *allium* family, is particularly good for the immune system.

SERVES 6–8
PREPARATION: about 30 minutes, plus overnight soaking
COOKING: about 2½ hours

225 g/8 oz dried cannellini beans
4 tablespoons olive oil
2 onions, finely chopped
2 leeks, finely chopped
2 carrots, chopped
2 celery stalks, chopped
400 g/14 oz tinned plum tomatoes
115 g/4 oz cavolo nero or cabbage, shredded
1 red chilli pepper
1 teaspoon chopped fresh oregano or ½ teaspoon dried
1 teaspoon chopped fresh rosemary or ½ teaspoon dried
2 litres/3½ pints miso broth (see page 176) or good-quality vegetable stock (see page 177)
100 ml/3½ fl oz dry white wine (optional)
Freshly ground sea salt and black pepper
8 thin slices of good-quality crusty wholemeal bread
4 garlic cloves
1 teaspoon chopped fresh thyme or ½ teaspoon dried
1 red onion, thinly sliced
55 g/2 oz Parmesan cheese, freshly grated

Soak the beans in water to cover generously and leave overnight.

Next day, drain and rinse the beans well. In a large heavy-based pan, heat 2 tablespoons of the oil and sauté the onion in it briefly until just translucent, then add the vegetables, chilli pepper, oregano and rosemary. Sauté for about 5 minutes, until all the vegetables are well coated in the oil and beginning to soften. Add the beans and mix in to coat them well.

Add the miso broth or stock and the wine. Bring to the boil, lower the heat and simmer for about 1½ hours, until the beans are quite soft. Season to taste (don't add salt before this point or the beans' skins will harden). Allow to cool slightly and fish out the chilli pepper.

Preheat the oven to 180°C/350°F/Gas 4. Ladle out about half the contents of the pan (try to favour the beans and leave the vegetables) and purée in a food processor or by means of a food mill. Return to the pan and mix well.

Rub the bread with one or two garlic cloves, toast lightly and set aside. Finely chop the remaining garlic. Heat the remaining oil in a frying pan and gently sauté the garlic with the thyme and lots of black pepper, until softened and aromatic. Stir this into the soup and adjust the seasoning if necessary.

Pour about half the pan's contents into an ovenproof casserole, spread the toasted bread over that and then empty the rest of the pan's contents on top. Arrange the slices of red onion over the top and scatter with the cheese.

Bake in the oven for about 30 minutes, until the top is golden.

CARROT AND CORIANDER SOUP

P ★★★★   E ★   A ★★★★

Carrot and coriander is a favourite combination for many people – and rightly so. They complement each other beautifully.

The many phytoestrogens in this recipe originate from a number of sources: the miso broth, tofu cream or soya yoghurt, soya milk and garlic. The carrots contain excellent amounts of the powerful antioxidant, beta-carotene, which is effective in delaying ageing and preventing cancer. The onion is especially useful for bone protection.

Water, miso broth or vegetable stock can be used as a base for the soup; obviously, if you use broth or stock it will have a deeper flavour, but the soup is still delicious made with just water.

SERVES 4
PREPARATION: about 20 minutes
COOKING: about 40 minutes

500g/1lb 2oz baby carrots, chopped small

1 large onion, chopped small

2 garlic cloves

Grated zest and juice of 1 uncoated orange

1 teaspoon ground coriander seeds

Large handful of coriander, with roots, plus more sprigs to garnish

600ml/1 pint boiling water, miso broth (see page 176) or vegetable stock (see page 177)

300ml/½ pint soya milk

Freshly ground sea salt and black pepper

2 teaspoons honey

100ml/3½ floz tofu cream (see page 183), thick unset plain yoghurt, preferably soya yoghurt, or whipping cream (optional)

Put the carrots, onion, garlic, orange zest and ground coriander in a large heavy pan with the coriander stalks and roots tied together by a couple of stalks. Add the water, broth or stock and soya milk, and bring to a simmer. Cook gently for about 30 minutes until everything is quite tender.

Transfer to a food processor or blender with most of the coriander leaves and the orange juice, and blitz to a purée. Pour and spoon back into the rinsed-out pan, taste and adjust the seasoning with salt, pepper and honey.

Stir in the tofu cream, yoghurt or cream, if using it, and heat through gently, stirring. Scatter over the reserved coriander leaves before serving.

THAI MUSHROOM NOODLE SOUP

P ★★★★   E ★★   A ★

Shiitake mushrooms are native to the Far East and are usually used in their dried form. In addition to the good phytoestrogen content of the mushroom family, shiitake mushrooms have been shown to carry other health benefits, including protection against both heart disease and cancer.

Phytoestrogens are also present in the tofu, beansprouts, miso broth and the garlic. Ginger is excellent for increasing the circulation and has traditionally been used for reducing inflammation in the joints and helping arthritis. It can also help with nausea, which some menopausal women complain of.

Hot and sour tom yum soup paste is now available in better supermarkets and good delis and health food stores. This pounded mixture of soya beans, lemon grass, Thai shallots, chillies, garlic and shrimp paste gives an instant Thai flavour to any soup. (See photograph opposite.)

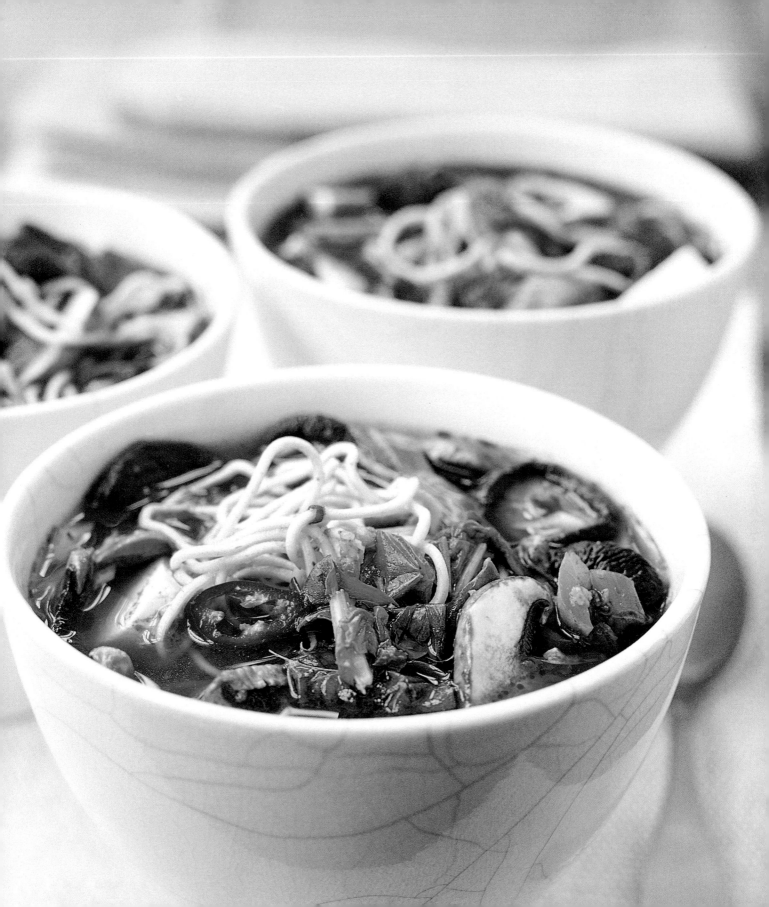

SERVES 4

PREPARATION: about 25 minutes,
plus 10 minutes' soaking

COOKING: about 20 minutes

25g/1oz dried shiitake or other mushrooms

150ml/¼ pint boiling water

175g/6oz fresh chestnut mushrooms

Bunch of spring onions

1.1 litres/2 pints miso broth (see page 176)

2 tablespoons tom yum soup paste

1 tablespoon soy sauce

½ small red chilli, thinly sliced (optional)

*2.5-cm/1-in piece of root ginger, peeled
and grated*

2 garlic cloves, thinly sliced

2 tablespoons no-added-sugar fish sauce

85g/3oz egg thread noodles

175g/6oz spinach or beansprouts, shredded

200g/7oz tofu, diced

First soak the dried mushrooms in the boiling water
for about 10 minutes. Drain them, reserving the
liquid. Then slice the chestnut mushrooms and
spring onions.

Bring the miso broth and reserved mushroom
liquid almost to the boil, then stir in the tom yum
soup paste. Add the sliced mushrooms, reserved
shiitake mushrooms, spring onions, soy sauce, chilli
(if using), ginger, garlic and fish sauce. Simmer for
about 10 minutes.

Add the noodles, spinach and tofu to the soup,
and cook for a further 3–5 minutes, until the
noodles are just tender.

To serve, divide the soup and noodles between
warmed serving bowls.

GUACAMOLE

P ★   E ★★   A ★★★★

Avocado is a wonderful fruit but it has been
given a bad name amongst slimmers because it
is high in calories. In fact, its calories come in
the form of the beneficial monounsaturated fats,
which are exceptionally easy to digest. Avocados
are high in potassium, the mineral that helps
prevent water retention, and are also a rich
source of vitamin E as well as vitamin C, B6,
riboflavin and manganese. They have also been
found to help produce collagen, which gives the
elasticity to skin and is essential for maintaining
strong bones.

The limes likewise contain good amounts of
vitamin C, which helps to increase the collagen
matrix in the bones. Spring onions are useful for
the bones and tomatoes contain the antioxidant
lycopene, which helps counter cell damage and
premature ageing.

It is traditional to serve this Mexican dip with
corn chips, but it is just as nice – and healthier –
accompanied by vegetable crudités. Whenever
they are available, try to use the black-skinned
Hass avocados, as they are more likely to be ripe
and tasty.

SERVES 4

PREPARATION: 15 minutes

4 spring onions

Large handful of coriander leaves

Grated zest and juice of 2 limes

3 large ripe avocados

2 small red chillies, deseeded and thinly sliced

*500g/1lb 2oz very ripe tomatoes, skinned (see page 50),
stalk ends removed and finely chopped*

Freshly ground sea salt and black pepper

Coarsely chop the spring onions into the bowl of a food processor and add all but a few sprigs of the coriander, the zest and juice of the limes, and the flesh of two of the avocados. Whizz to a purée.

Add the remaining avocado, the chilli and all but a few spoonfuls of the tomatoes and pulse gently until the avocado flesh is broken up but there are still visible small chunks of it. Do not over-process. Season generously to taste with salt and pepper.

Pour into serving bowls, spoon a little of the reserved chopped tomato into the centre of each bowl and top with a reserved coriander leaf.

HUMMUS BI TAHINI

P ★★★★★   E ★★★★★   A ★★

This is one of my favourite dishes for the menopause because it is tasty and yet extremely good for us. Chickpeas are a very good source of phytoestrogens because they contain all four isoflavones. The olives and olive oil are good for lowering cholesterol and helping the heart. The sesame seeds in the tahini contain high amounts of calcium and essential fatty acids. To increase the EFA content further, drizzle some olive oil and linseed oil over the hummus at the end.

Tahini paste can easily be made at home by puréeing sesame seeds. Hummus, the chickpea purée, is so frequently mixed with tahini that this mixture is itself often simply called hummus. As well as being a delicious starter and dip with pitta or rye bread, it also makes a wonderful sauce for barbecued or roast vegetables or fish. It is so rich in nutritional goodies that it should also be favoured as a savoury snack (it's great on oatcakes) – if you want to boost the phyto content even further, sprinkle it with some lightly toasted pine nuts.

SERVES 6–8

PREPARATION: about 15 minutes, plus overnight soaking if using dried chickpeas

COOKING: about 1 hour (if using dried chickpeas)

450g/1lb chickpeas or 2 large (400g/14oz) tins of cooked chickpeas, drained

4 large garlic cloves

2 hot red chillies

Juice of about 3 lemons

About 150ml/¼ pint tahini paste

85g/3oz pitted black olives, plus a few for garnish

2 teaspoons ground cumin

About 1 teaspoon freshly ground sea salt

Extra-virgin olive oil, to dress

A little paprika, to garnish

Chopped flat-leaved parsley, to garnish

Warm pitta bread, to serve

If using dried chickpeas, soak them overnight in water. Next day, discard the water, cover with fresh cold water and bring to the boil. Lower the heat, add one of the garlic cloves and the chillies and simmer for 1 hour, until just soft. Drain, reserving the water and discarding the garlic and chillies.

Reserving a few whole chickpeas, put the rest in a food processor with the lemon juice, tahini paste, olives, cumin, 150ml/¼ pint of the reserved water (or plain water or miso broth, see page 176, if using tinned chickpeas) and salt. Chop the remaining garlic, add to the processor and blitz to a coarse purée. The consistency should not be too smooth, with discernible pieces of chickpeas giving texture. Add more water if too dry. Adjust the flavouring with more tahini, lemon juice and salt to taste.

Spread the hummus on individual plates, forking circular ridges on the surface. Pour a little olive oil over and arrange a few whole chickpeas and olives on top, dust with a little paprika and garnish with the flat-leaved parsley. Serve with warm pitta bread.

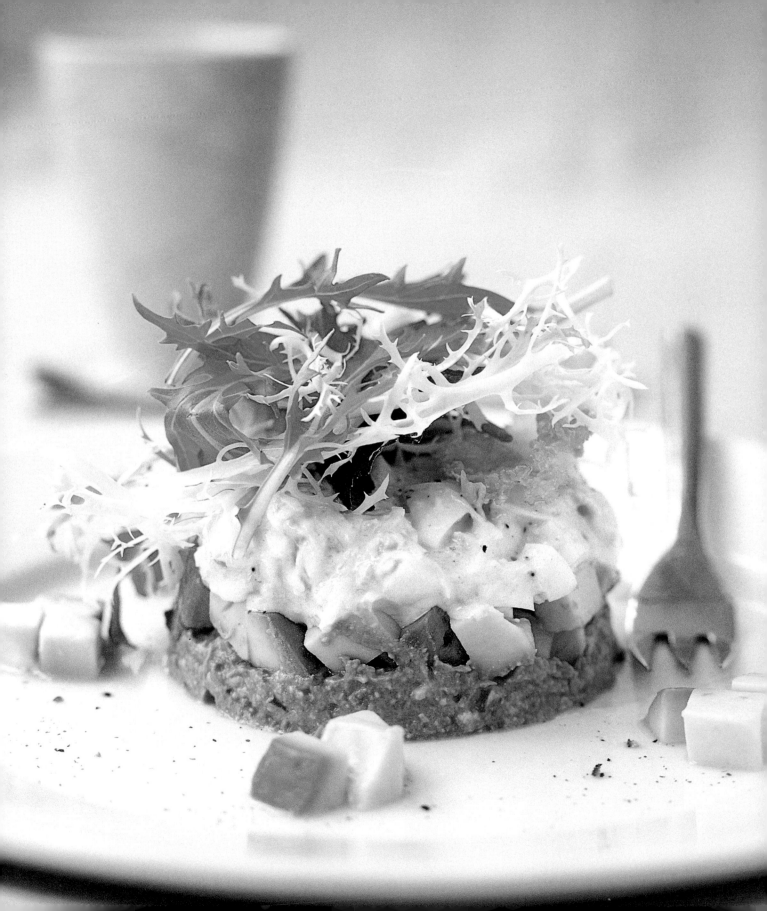

CRAB AND AVOCADO SALAD

P ★★★   E ★★★   A ★★★

This delicately flavoured salad (see photograph opposite) supplies good amounts of antioxidants via both the avocado and the crab. Crab contains zinc and magnesium as well as selenium, which is anti-ageing and cancer-protective. It is also a good source of essential fatty acids, which are important for lubricating the skin and vagina as well as the joints.

Avocados have been shown to help produce collagen, which is important for maintaining healthy skin and bones. They also have high amounts of the mineral potassium, which helps prevent water retention. Linseeds are an excellent source of phytoestrogen and provide essential fatty acids.

SERVES 4
PREPARATION: about 15 minutes
COOKING: 10 minutes (for the egg)

1 large avocado, preferably Hass
Juice of 1 lemon
200g/7oz dressed fresh crab meat (brown and white)
½ teaspoon anchovy paste
½ teaspoon mustard powder
2 tablespoons golden linseeds
Freshly ground sea salt and black pepper
2 large eggs, hard-boiled, shelled and chopped
3 tablespoons mayonnaise (ready-made or see page 179)
Mixed soft salad leaves, to serve

Peel, halve, stone and dice the avocado. Toss the pieces in the juice of half the lemon.

Pick over the crab meat to remove any residual pieces of shell. Put the brown meat in one bowl and flake the white into another. Into the brown meat, mix the remaining lemon juice, the anchovy paste, mustard powder and linseeds, with seasoning to taste. Into the white flesh, gently mix the egg and the mayonnaise with any remaining lemon juice drained from the avocado and some seasoning. Arrange the salad leaves on serving plates. There are two ways of serving this: either combine the contents of both bowls together with the avocado dice and spoon mounds of this on top of the salad; or arrange in layers, with the avocado on top of the leaves, followed by the brown meat and then the white. Layering inside a round pastry cutter helps give a neat and attractive shape.

SALADE NICOISE

P ★★   E ★★★★★   A ★★★

Apart from being a sophisticated and delicious salad, this dish is supremely good for your well-being. Healthy servings of phytoestrogens are provided by the potatoes, green beans and herbs – especially if you choose parsley and sage. The salad dressing holds extra phytoestrogens in the garlic. Good quantities of monounsaturated oils are available from the black olives as well as the olive oil in the dressing. The eggs are an excellent healthy source of protein and are packed with nutrients, especially the B vitamins (the 'anti-stress' vitamins) and zinc (essential for hormone balance and healthy bones). Essential fatty acids in the form of Omega 3 are contained in the anchovies and to a lesser degree in the tuna.

SERVES 4–6
PREPARATION: 20 minutes
COOKING: 15–20 minutes (for the potatoes and eggs)

225g/8oz small new potatoes

175g/6oz fine green beans

2–3 eggs

1 Cos lettuce or 2 Little Gems

Small bunch of spring onions

½ cucumber

225g/8oz tomatoes

1 red pepper

1 large tin (200g/7oz) of tuna chunks in oil

About 100g/3½oz anchovy fillets, rinsed and drained

115g/4oz pitted black olives, preferably garlic-flavoured

Several handfuls of fresh herbs, particularly flat-leaved parsley, chives, basil, chervil and tarragon

FOR THE DRESSING:

1 garlic clove

3 tablespoons extra-virgin olive oil

2 tablespoons linseed oil

1 tablespoon balsamic vinegar

Freshly ground sea salt and black pepper

Put a pan of salted water on to heat. Scrub the potatoes or peel only if absolutely necessary. When the water is boiling, add the beans and blanch for 1–2 minutes only. Remove with a slotted spoon and drop into a bowl of cold water.

Add the potatoes to the boiling water and cook them at a good simmer until barely tender – they must not become mushy. Put another pan of water on to heat and add the eggs. They should be boiled for 12 minutes only and no more.

While the potatoes and eggs are cooking, prepare the other fresh vegetables. Shred the lettuce leaves into the bottom of a large salad bowl. Trim the spring onions and snip them over the leaves. Slice the cucumber lengthwise into 2 or 3 long slices and then cut these into long strips; finally cut across into 2-cm/¾-in chunks. Quarter the tomatoes and halve these quarters again if large. Halve and deseed the pepper and slice the flesh across into thinnish strips. Add all these to the bowl.

Drain the tuna and flake in half of it at this stage. Using scissors, snip in half the anchovies and add half the olives. Snip in half the herbs.

By this time the potatoes should be cooked and the eggs hard-boiled. Drain and dry the potatoes briefly over a very low heat, then leave to cool slightly on a flat plate. Drain the eggs and dunk them in cold water. Pour off the water from the cooled beans and drain on paper towels.

Make the dressing: crush the garlic into the mixed oils, add the vinegar and season with salt and pepper to taste. Mix well until a smooth emulsion and adjust the seasoning.

Cut the potatoes into bite-sized chunks if necessary and add these to the salad, together with the beans. Pour the dressing over the salad, toss well to mix. At this stage taste and adjust the seasoning.

Shell the eggs, cut into quarters and arrange over the top of the salad, together with the remaining tuna, olives and anchovies. Snip over the herbs.

PIEDMONTESE PEPPERS WITH ANCHOVIES

P ★★   E ★★★   A ★★★★

This dish (see photograph opposite) not only makes a lovely starter, but is also excellent in helping different aspects of the menopause. Phytoestrogens are included in the form of the garlic and peppers, and help prevent cancer and premature ageing. Peppers can contain twice as much vitamin C as oranges – which may come as a surprise to some people. Vitamin C is vital for the bones as it produces collagen, which makes up some 90 per cent of the bone matrix.

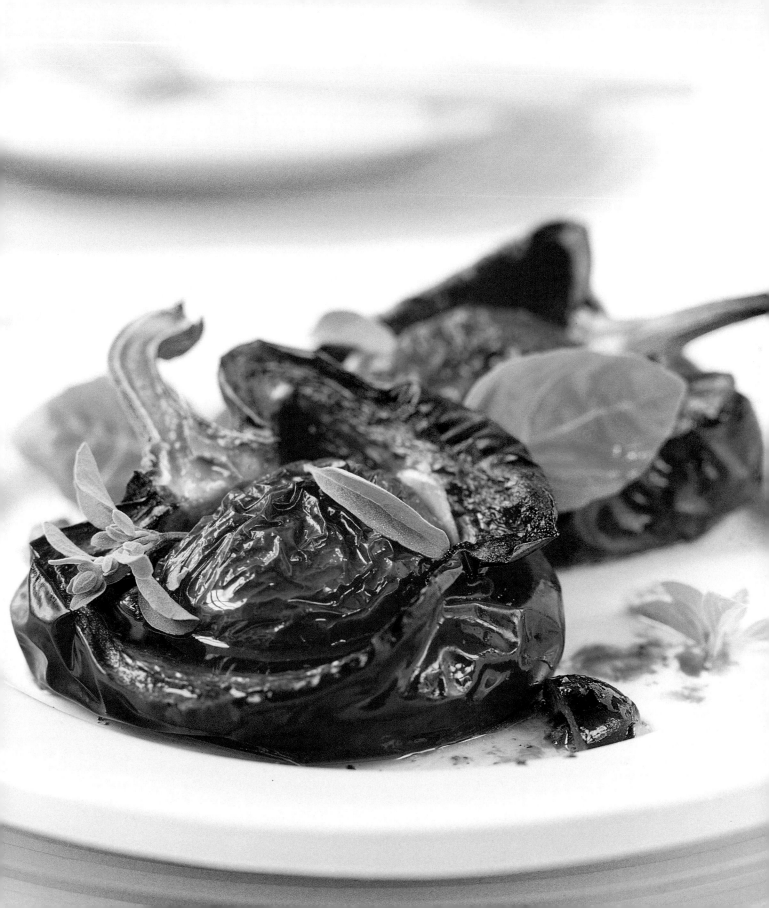

The anchovies contain essential fatty acids in the form of Omega 3 oils, which help to lubricate the joints and keep the skin and vagina soft and pliable. These oils can also reduce the risk of heart disease. The herb basil is noted for its tranquillising effect on the body – important at the menopause when our moods can fluctuate – and oregano is good for the digestion.

SERVES 4
PREPARATION: 10 minutes
COOKING: 25–30 minutes

4 red or yellow peppers
4 garlic cloves, sliced
50g/2oz pitted black olives, chopped
4 anchovy fillets, rinsed, drained and chopped
1 tablespoon capers, rinsed and drained
4 plum tomatoes, halved
3 tablespoons extra-virgin olive oil, plus more for greasing
Freshly ground sea salt and black pepper
Large handful of fresh basil, roughly chopped
2 tablespoons fresh oregano, roughly chopped

Preheat the oven to 220°C/425°F/Gas 7. Halve the peppers and remove the seeds but not the stalks. Place the peppers skin-side down on a lightly oiled baking sheet.

Place slices of garlic inside each pepper half, scatter with the olive and anchovy pieces and the capers, then top each with a plum tomato half, cut-side down. Drizzle with the oil, season and bake for 10 minutes.

Reduce the oven setting to 200°C/400°F/Gas 6 and continue baking for a further 15–20 minutes, until the peppers and tomatoes are tender.

Serve the peppers hot or cold, scattered with the fresh herbs.

MOROCCAN CARROT AND ORANGE SALAD

P ★★★   E ★★★   A ★★★★★

You could call this the Moroccan Antioxidant Salad just from its glorious colour: it is full of beta-carotene, which is particularly strong in orange fruits and vegetables. The carrots also contain good amounts of phytoestrogens, as do the linseeds, which are rich in essential fatty acids too.

As well as being an ideal summer starter, this salad makes a fine accompaniment to spicy vegetable and grain dishes and strongly flavoured fish dishes. You could also toss in a few cubes of tofu to create an excellent light meal or snack. Adding tofu to the salad would mean that the phytoestrogen content is increased from ★★★ to ★★★★. (See photograph, page 16.)

SERVES 4
PREPARATION: 10 minutes, plus chilling

2 large juicy navel oranges
350g/12oz baby carrots
1 head of chicory
Pinch of cinnamon or 1 tablespoon orange flower water (optional)

FOR THE DRESSING:
1 tablespoon clear honey
2 tablespoons extra-virgin olive oil
1 tablespoon linseed oil
1 tablespoon golden linseeds
1 tablespoon lemon juice
2 tablespoons coriander, finely chopped (optional)
Freshly ground sea salt and black pepper

Peel the orange, removing as much of the white pith as you can. Using a sharp knife, slice the fruit horizontally into very thin round slices and then cut these in half, reserving the resulting juices for the dressing.

Scrub the carrots and pare them into long shreds. Trim the chicory of its base and discard the outer leaves. Separate the inner leaves. Place the shredded carrots, chicory leaves and orange slices in a salad bowl. Chill briefly.

Just before serving, beat the dressing ingredients together with the reserved orange juice until they are well blended. Season to taste. Pour the dressing over the salad and toss carefully until well coated. Sprinkle over some cinnamon or orange flower water if you like.

Variation: this salad is also good sprinkled with some lightly toasted pine nuts.

MUSHROOM CROSTINI

P ★★   E ★   A ★

This irresistible starter smells and tastes luxurious, with its combination of garlic, mushrooms, herbs and olive oil.

All these are good for you, in various ways. For instance, the two members of the *allium* family – garlic and shallots – are excellent for the immune system and the garlic is particularly effective against tumours. Phytoestrogens are contained in the mushrooms, sage, garlic, parsley and bread.

SERVES 4
PREPARATION: 15 minutes,
plus 20 minutes' soaking
COOKING: about 25 minutes

40g/1½oz dried porcini mushrooms

1 tablespoon olive oil

Knob of butter

2 shallots, finely chopped

2 garlic cloves, crushed

1 teaspoon finely chopped fresh sage

Dash of balsamic vinegar

150g/5oz chestnut mushrooms

Small handful of flat-leaved parsley, plus more to garnish

Freshly ground sea salt and black pepper

1 ciabatta loaf, cut into 4 lengths and each piece cut across in half

Rinse the dried mushrooms carefully in cold running water, then put them to soak in a small bowl of warm water for about 20 minutes. Lift them out, pat them dry and chop them coarsely. Sieve the soaking water and set aside.

Heat the oil with the butter in a wide-based pan and sauté the shallots until translucent. Add the garlic, sauté briefly until aromatic, then add the reconstituted mushrooms with 150½ml/½ pint of the strained soaking liquid plus the sage and vinegar. Cover and cook over a gentle heat for about 15 minutes.

In the meantime, wipe the fresh mushrooms clean with paper towels. Slice them not too thinly. Turn the heat up and add them to the pan with the parsley, reserving a few sprigs for garnish. Cook over a moderate to high heat for 5–7 minutes uncovered, stirring occasionally, until most of the liquid has evaporated. Season to taste.

Toast the slices of bread and spread a generous layer of the mushroom mixture on top. Serve immediately, garnished with the reserved parsley.

Variation: make this into a more substantial snack by adding a layer of cheese, such as Mozzarella or grated Parmesan.

PRAWN AND SESAME TOASTS

P ★   E ★★   A ★

Prawns are a good source of vitamin B12 as well
as the important mineral selenium, which is a
powerful antioxidant and beneficial in
preventing cancer and ageing. The wholemeal
bread provides phytoestrogens, as do the sesame
seeds and parsley, if used. As this is a fried dish,
keep it for special treats only.

Buy fresh firm prawns for this dish. Rinse
them well and pat them quite dry with paper
towels. If using frozen prawns, make sure they
are well defrosted and drained – you will also
need about twice the weight of fresh prawns, as
once their ice glaze melts away you will be
surprised at how little is left.

SERVES 4 (makes about 48)
PREPARATION: 10 minutes
COOKING: 15–20 minutes

4 spring onions
225 g / 8 oz cooked prawns, peeled
*Small sprig of coriander, plus more leaves
to garnish (optional)*
*2-cm / ¾-in piece of fresh root ginger, peeled and
crushed in a garlic press*
2 teaspoons cornflour
½ teaspoon honey
2 teaspoons light soy sauce
1 teaspoon dry sherry
Good dash of Tabasco (optional)
½ teaspoon dark sesame oil
1 egg

Freshly ground sea salt and black pepper
Olive oil, for frying
12 thin slices of day-old wholemeal bread, crusts removed
4 tablespoons sesame seeds
Lime wedges, to serve (optional)

Coarsely snip the spring onions into the bowl of a
food processor. Add the prawns, coriander, ginger
(all the juice and bits included), cornflour, honey,
soy sauce, sherry, Tabasco to taste (if using) and the
sesame oil and whizz until the spring onions and
prawns are finely chopped.

Add the egg, season generously with salt and
pepper to taste and whizz again briefly until the
mixture forms a smoothish paste.

Pour the olive oil into a wok or large frying pan
to a depth of about 1cm/½ in and heat to the point
where a small cube of the bread will brown in about
40 seconds.

While the oil is heating, spread each slice of bread
with some of the prawn mixture. Sprinkle the tops
with sesame seeds.

Cut each slice of bread into 4 triangles or long
strips. Fry the strips in batches, paste side down, for
about 1 minute and then turn them over and fry the
other side very briefly (about 15–20 seconds), until
the toasts are a uniform golden brown. As soon as
each batch is cooked, remove from the pan, drain
them on layers of paper towels and keep in a warm
place, uncovered.

Serve as soon as all are cooked with lime wedges
on the side and garnished with some more
coriander if you wish.

Variations: Vary the flavour of the prawn mixture
by using parsley instead of coriander and/or
replacing the ginger with some chopped seaweed.

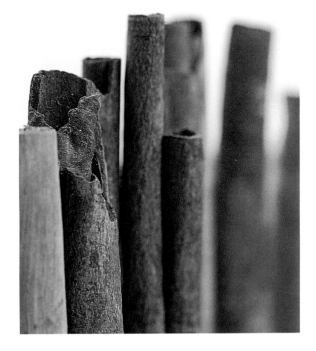

Breakfasts
and
brunches

KEDGEREE

P ★★★★★   E ★★   A ★★★★

An excellent variety of phytoestrogens are contained in this one dish, from the soya milk, soya cream, lentils, brown rice and cinnamon through to the parsley. The spices benefit the digestive system: cumin is traditionally known to help counter flatulence, cardamom is used to aid digestion and cayenne acts as a general tonic for the digestive system.

If you want to serve this comforting breakfast dish for brunch, you can give it more of a savoury punch by frying one or two sliced onions with a couple of garlic cloves until crisp. Mix these in or sprinkle them over the top.

SERVES 4–6
PREPARATION: 15 minutes
COOKING: about 25 minutes

225 g/8 oz brown basmati rice

225 g/8 oz split red lentils

About 450 g/1 lb undyed smoked haddock

About 150 ml/¼ pint soya milk

1–2 bay leaves

1 cinnamon stick

4–5 black peppercorns

6 cardamom pods

1 lime, plus more to serve (optional)

Large handful of flat-leaved parsley, plus more to garnish

Large handful of coriander, plus more to garnish

3–4 tablespoons soya cream

Pinch of ground cumin

Freshly ground sea salt and black pepper

Pinch or two of cayenne pepper

2–3 hard-boiled eggs, cut into wedges

First put the rice and lentils to soak in a large bowl, covered generously with water.

Rinse the haddock well under cold running water and put it in a pan with soya milk barely to cover (cut the fish into manageable pieces if necessary). Add a bay leaf or two, half the cinnamon stick and the black peppercorns and bring to the boil. Poach gently for 2–4 minutes, until the fish is stiff and beginning to flake (the exact time will depend on how thick it is). Drain and let the fish cool a little.

When the fish is cool enough to handle, flake it into a bowl, taking some care to remove any remaining bones.

Put a large pan of lightly salted water on to boil. Lightly crush the cardamom pods and add to the water with the rest of the cinnamon. Drain the soaking rice and lentils into a sieve and rinse thoroughly under cold running water until the water runs clear.

Tip the rice and lentils into the heating water and bring to the boil. Stir, cover and cook until both the rice and lentils are just tender, 20–30 minutes depending on variety and age.

When the rice and lentils are ready, drain thoroughly. Return to the pan and fish out the pieces of cinnamon and cardamom (they will probably all gather in one place). Place over a very low heat and fork the rice once or twice to help it dry off.

Grate in the zest of the lime and pour in the juice. Snip in most of the parsley and coriander. Add the soya cream with the cumin stirred into it. Stir well over a moderate heat to warm everything through and then add the fish. Season to taste with salt, pepper and cayenne.

Turn out into a warmed serving dish, dot all over with the wedges of hard-boiled egg and garnish with the reserved flat-leaved parsley and a few coriander leaves.

Serve with lime wedges, if you like.

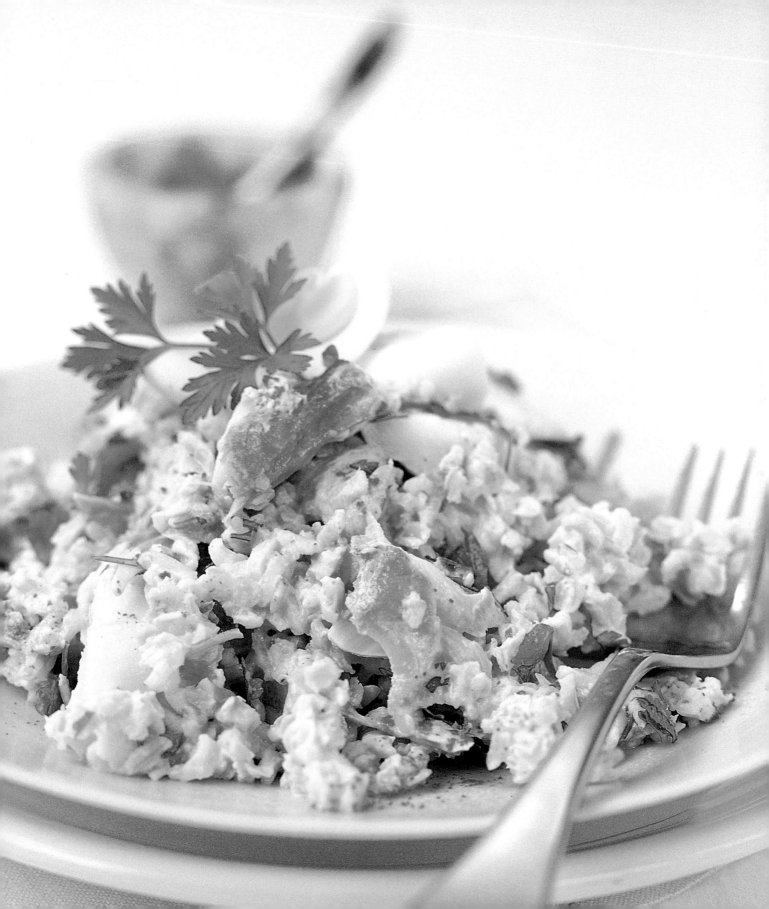

PAPAYA WITH SMOKED FISH MOUSSE

P ★★★   E ★★★   A ★

With its bright colours, this is a very pretty dish as well as having a wonderful flavour. Mackerel is very good for the health because of its high levels of essential fatty acids in the form of Omega 3 oils. The soya cream provides phytoestrogens in good supply.

SERVES 4–6
PREPARATION: about 10 minutes

2 papayas

1 lime

FOR THE MOUSSE:

350g/12oz smoked mackerel fillets, skinned

150ml/¼ pint soya cream

Juice of 1 lime, plus more if necessary

Freshly ground sea salt and black pepper

1–2 tablespoon(s) horseradish cream

Tabasco sauce

First make the mousse: flake the fish into a large bowl and add the soya cream and lime juice. Using a fork, mix well to a smoothish purée. Season with salt and pepper, horseradish, Tabasco and more lime juice to taste.

Halve the papayas, scoop out the seeds and then peel off the skins. You can then either serve the mousse spooned into the cavities (take a little sliver off the base of each papaya half so they will sit stably) or slice each half almost all the way across lengthwise, fan it out and set the mousse alongside. Either way, squeeze lime juice over all the papaya flesh to prevent discoloration, and sprinkle with some pepper.

PORTUGUESE OMELETTE

P ★★   E ★   A ★

Designed for the developing chick, eggs are an excellent source of nutrients. Although high in cholesterol, they are low in saturated fat. Egg yolk is rich in lecithin, which transports fat in the blood and can help prevent the build-up of plaque in the arteries. This lowers the risk of heart disease, which is a particular risk during and after the menopause. Phytoestrogens are in the parsley and the wholewheat of the croûtons. Cayenne is good for the digestive system.

SERVES 1

PREPARATION: about 15 minutes, plus making the croûtons

COOKING: about 5 minutes

Handful of cold garlic croûtons (see page 52)

2 tablespoons Parmesan cheese, grated

1 tablespoon parsley, chopped

Pinch of cayenne pepper

2 large eggs

Dash of no-added-sugar Worcestershire sauce

Freshly ground sea salt and black pepper

Large knob of butter or 1 tablespoon olive oil

1 tablespoon poppy seeds

1 teaspoon linseeds

First put the croûtons in a plastic bag with the Parmesan, parsley and cayenne, and shake well until they are thoroughly coated.

In a bowl, lightly beat the eggs with the Worcestershire sauce and some seasoning to taste.

Melt the butter or oil in an omelette pan over a moderate heat and, when it foams, add the eggs. Using a fork, pull the edges of the omelette into the centre as they cook until there is a nice pile of softly cooked curds in the centre and still some runny egg around that, but the underside is firm and browned. Sprinkle the croûtons, poppy seeds and linseeds over one half of the omelette and fold the other half over that. Slide the omelette out on to a warmed plate.

FRENCH TOAST

P ★★   E ★   A ★

You can use all types of bread for French toast, or *pain perdu* (lost bread), as long as it is old enough to be dryish, or it will absorb too much of the egg and fall apart on cooking. Try it with wholemeal bread, brioche or challah, sliced baguette or even croissants. It is delicious topped with maple syrup, fruit compôte (see page 79) or soft fruit like raspberries and blueberries.

This dish should really be kept as a treat, although the soya milk and wholemeal bread give a good helping of phytoestrogens.

SERVES 8
PREPARATION: about 10 minutes
COOKING: 10–20 minutes

4 eggs
Pinch of freshly ground sea salt
225 ml/8 fl oz soya milk
½ teaspoon vanilla extract
½ teaspoon ground cinnamon, plus more to serve
Butter or olive oil, for greasing
8 slices slightly stale bread (see above)
Maple syrup, dried fruit compôte (see page 79) or fresh berries, to serve

In a bowl, beat the eggs lightly and add the salt, soya milk, vanilla and cinnamon. Beat again until frothy.

Grease a griddle pan lightly with butter or oil and get it hot. Dip each slice of bread into the egg mixture until it is well coated and cook on the hot griddle pan until well browned on both sides (you may have to do this in batches and keep warm).

Serve sprinkled with more cinnamon and some maple syrup, fruit compôte or berries.

Variation: try adding the grated zest and juice of 1 large orange to the egg mixture.

SCRAMBLED TOFU

P ★★★★   E ★   A ★

A wonderful way to start the day, the tofu and parsley in the dish are packed full of phytoestrogens. Serve with wholemeal bread or toast, or with grilled tomatoes.

SERVES 4
PREPARATION: about 10 minutes
COOKING: 6–8 minutes

1 tablespoon fresh basil, shredded, or 1 teaspoon dried basil
2 tablespoons flat-leaved parsley, finely chopped
1 tablespoon soy sauce
2 teaspoons olive oil
2 spring onions, chopped
225 g/8 oz soft tofu, crumbled

In a bowl or using a mortar and pestle, mash together the basil, parsley and soy sauce. Set aside.

Heat the oil in a pan and, when hot, sauté the spring onions until just wilted. Stir in the tofu followed by the herb mixture and stir-fry for another 3–4 minutes.

FRITTATA FOO YUNG

P ★ ★ ★   E ★ ★   A ★ ★ ★

This is an excellent recipe for its phytoestrogen content due to the soya cream and bean spouts, the one a source of isoflavones, the other coumestans. The olive oil is a good monounsaturated fat which can help reduce cholesterol and so maintain a healthy heart.

The prawns are low in saturated fat and high in protein. They are also an excellent source of vitamin B12 and a good source of the mineral selenium, which acts as a powerful antioxidant in the fight against cancer and helps prevent premature ageing.

Ginger has traditionally been used for easing joint pains and arthritis as it can reduce inflammation. It is also used to help circulation and digestion.

Celery also has anti-inflammatory properties and contains good amounts of potassium, which helps to alleviate water retention – often a source of weight gain at the menopause. Another source of phytoestrogen, celery is commonly used in Eastern medicine to treat high blood pressure, a remedy which has recently been confirmed in the West.

SERVES 4
PREPARATION: 10 minutes
COOKING: about 10 minutes

6 eggs
Freshly ground sea salt and black pepper
3 tablespoons soya cream
2 teaspoons soy sauce, plus more for dressing
2 tablespoons olive oil
2–3 thin slices of root ginger, finely chopped
1 celery heart stalk, thinly sliced
6 spring onions, chopped
200g/7oz beansprouts
1 tablespoon linseeds
85g/3oz cooked peeled small prawns
A few chive stalks, to garnish (optional)

Preheat a hot grill. Break the eggs into a large bowl and beat well until quite frothy. Season lightly with salt and well with pepper and stir in the soya cream. Add the soy sauce and mix well.

Heat half the oil in a wok or large frying pan and, when hot, stir-fry the ginger, celery and spring onions until just wilted. Then add in the beansprouts, linseeds and prawns, toss to coat and heat through well – but make sure you do not overcook. Set aside and keep warm.

Brush the bottom and sides of a medium-sized heatproof frying pan with the remaining oil and place over a moderate to high heat. As soon as the oil gets hot, stir the egg mixture well again and tip it into the pan.

Pull the edges of the solidifying egg into the centre two or three times and then immediately tip the stir-fried mixture on top of the eggs. Arrange uniformly over the top with a fork, pressing the filling ingredients into the egg, and continue to cook over a slightly reduced heat for about 3 minutes until it is firmly set on the base.

Put under the grill as close to the heat as you can get. Grill until the top is just browned and set. Serve cut into wedges, garnished with a few whole chive stalks and sprinkled with some more soy sauce if you like.

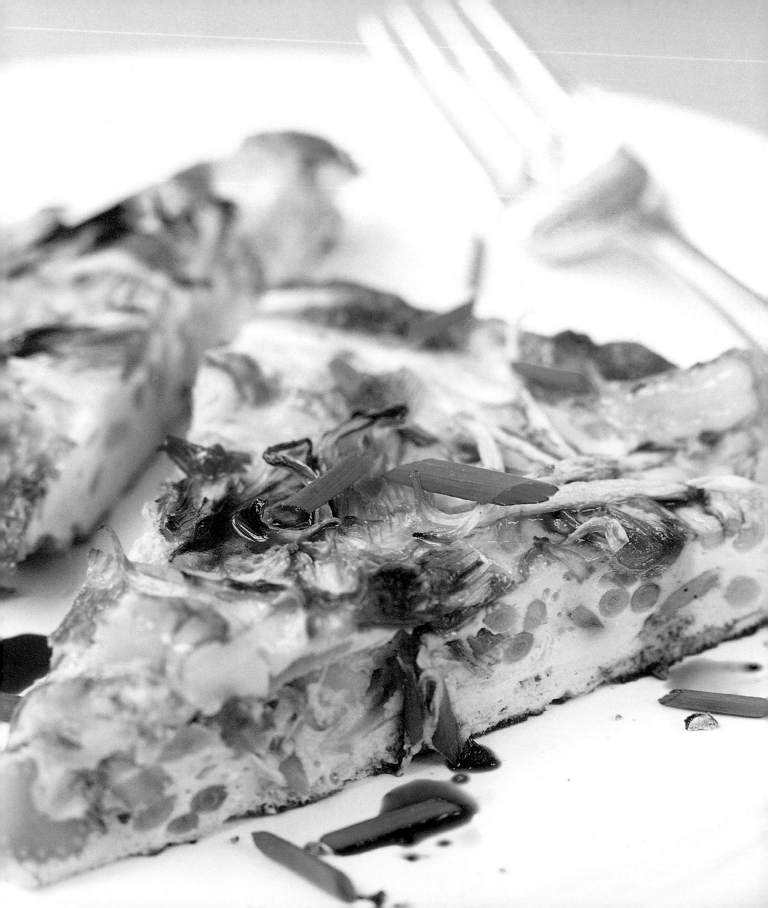

Eggs Florentine

P ★★★★   E ★   A ★

Eggs are good for the health in many ways. Although they have a bad name because of their high cholesterol content, they are low in saturated fat and a healthy source of protein. The egg yolk contains lecithin, which helps lower the risk of heart disease by preventing plaque from accumulating in the arteries.

Phytoestrogens are contained in good amounts in the soya flour and soya cream as well as the wholemeal bread.

SERVES 4
PREPARATION: about 20 minutes
COOKING: about 20 minutes

350g/12oz spinach, stalks removed
Freshly ground sea salt and black pepper
15g/½oz soya flour
2–3 tablespoons soya cream
Freshly grated nutmeg
4 slices of wholemeal bread
Butter or olive oil, for greasing and frying
A few drops of cider or red wine vinegar
4 very fresh eggs

FOR THE MORNAY SAUCE:
15g/½oz butter
2 tablespoons flour
300ml/½ pint soya milk
Freshly ground sea salt and black pepper
Freshly grated nutmeg
175g/6oz mature Cheddar cheese, grated

Put the spinach in a pan with only the water from washing it clinging to its leaves. Cover tightly and cook over a gentle heat for 2 minutes. Add a pinch of sea salt, cover again, increase the heat to moderate and cook for about 5 minutes more until the spinach is tender.

Drain very thoroughly, squeezing out any excess moisture with the back of a spoon, and return to the pan.

Mix the soya flour into the soya cream with nutmeg to taste and then combine this with the spinach. Simmer gently until thickened and no moisture runs from it when spooned to one side of the pan. Keep warm.

Preheat a hot grill and bring a pan of water to a simmer for the eggs.

Cut out rounds from the slices of bread big enough to line the bases of 4 large ramekins. Fry these in butter or olive oil until good and crisp on both sides.

While the croûtes are frying, make the Mornay sauce: melt the butter or oil in a heavy-based saucepan and stir in the flour. Cook over a moderate heat for a minute or two until the flour mixture just begins to colour. Then stir in the soya milk and whisk until smooth. Bring to the boil and simmer for about 5 minutes.

Season to taste with salt, pepper and nutmeg, and then stir in the Cheddar cheese. Check the flavouring and adjust the seasoning if necessary. Keep warm.

Add a few drops of vinegar to the simmering water and poach the eggs gently until opaque, a few minutes. Pour some cold water into the pan to stop the eggs from cooking, but leave them in the water to keep warm.

Using butter or olive oil, grease the sides of the ramekins, put the croûtes in the bottom and spoon the spinach mixture on top of that. Draining them well on a slotted spoon, set a poached egg on top of each, then pour over the Mornay sauce. Cook briefly under the hot grill, until bubbling. Serve at once.

MIDDLE-EASTERN PANCAKES

P ★★★   E ★★★   A ★

Phytoestrogens are present in the soya flour, soya milk, wholemeal flour and cinnamon. The culture in live organic yoghurt is excellent for intestinal health.

Almonds are a good source of essential fatty acids, the oils that we need to lubricate our joints and skin, and an excellent source of vitamin E, an antioxidant. Dates are high in magnesium ('nature's tranquilliser') as well as potassium, so useful in reducing water retention.

SERVES 4–6 (makes about 12)
**PREPARATION: 15 minutes,
plus 20 minutes' standing**
COOKING: about 30 minutes

FOR THE BATTER:

85 g/3 oz plain flour

25 g/1 oz soya flour

Pinch of freshly ground sea salt

150 ml/¼ pint natural yoghurt

1 egg

175 ml/6 fl oz soya milk

Finely grated zest of ½ lemon

FOR THE FILLING:

75 g/3 oz ground almonds

White of 1 egg, lightly beaten

1 tablespoon orange flower water

3 tablespoons date syrup

Finely grated zest of ½ lemon

2 teaspoons ground cinnamon

115 g/4 oz pitted dates, chopped

Butter or oil, for greasing and frying

FOR THE TOPPING:

Juice of 1 lemon

2 tablespoons date syrup

55 g/2 oz pistachios, chopped

First make the pancake batter: sieve the flours and salt into a large bowl. Make a well in the centre, add the yoghurt, break in the egg and beat until smooth. Gradually beat in the soya milk and then add the lemon zest. Allow to stand, covered, for about 20 minutes.

Make the filling: in a bowl, mix together the ground almonds, egg white, orange flower water and date syrup until smooth. Stir in the lemon zest, cinnamon and the dates.

Preheat a hot grill.

Lightly grease a 17.5-cm/7-in pancake pan with butter or oil and place over a high heat. When it is hot, reduce the heat to moderate and pour a tablespoon of batter into the pan. Tilt the pan to spread it all over the base of the pan. Cook for 1 minute, then flip the pancake over and fry the other side for the same time. Turn out on a sheet of baking paper and fold that over to keep it warm. Repeat with the rest of the batter, wiping and greasing the pan between each pancake. Pile the pancakes on top of one another, with a layer of baking paper between each.

Put a heaped spoonful of the filling in the centre of each pancake and fold it over, then fold in the ends and roll it up. Grease a heatproof dish just big enough to take the pancakes in a single layer and arrange them in it.

For the topping: stir the lemon juice in to the date syrup and spoon over the pancakes. Sprinkle with the pistachios and grill until the syrup is bubbling and the pancakes have darkened in colour slightly.

Serve with dollops of more yoghurt and a little date syrup.

BREAKFAST MUFFINS

P ★★★★★   E ★★   A ★★★★★

Muffins for breakfast may seem naughty, but this recipe is full of goodness, especially with the use of soya flour, soya milk and wholemeal flour. These are all good sources of phytoestrogens, as are the cinnamon, cranberries and the orange zest.

Blueberries and cranberries contain proanthocyanidins, which are excellent antioxidants and so play a major part in the prevention of heart disease and strokes. As they help to preserve the integrity of the capillaries they play a role in preventing varicose veins. The proanthocyanidins also contribute towards osteoporosis prevention because of their effect on collagen: by cross-linking collagen fibres, they strengthen the collagen matrix and stop its destruction.

Nuts and dried fruits are particularly rich in nutrients. Pecan nuts contain good amounts of essential fatty acids and the B vitamins and are often classed as 'calming foods'. Apricots are an excellent source of the antioxidant beta-carotene. What's more, the drying process increases levels of beta-carotene. Apricots also contain high levels of potassium, beneficial for reducing high blood pressure and water retention. Lastly, raisins supply good amounts of potassium and are low in fat.

These muffins are great on their own, and even tastier accompanied by butter with honey or sugar-free jam. They also make a good portable high-phyto snack for getting you through the day.

MAKES 12

PREPARATION: about 20 minutes

COOKING: 20–25 minutes, plus cooling

Olive oil for greasing
200g/7oz plain flour
3 tablespoons soya flour
Pinch of freshly ground sea salt
2 teaspoons baking powder
2 eggs
55g/2oz butter, melted
175ml/6floz soya milk
125ml/4½floz maple syrup
125g/4½oz fresh blueberries
125g/4½oz dried cranberries, chopped
125g/4½oz seedless raisins
125g/4½oz dried apricots, chopped
50g/2oz pecans, chopped
1 teaspoon grated orange zest
1 teaspoon ground cinnamon

Preheat the oven to 200°C/400°F/Gas 6 and, using olive oil, grease some muffin tins with 6-cm/2½-in diameter indentations.

Sift the flours, salt and baking powder into a bowl. In another bowl, lightly beat the eggs, then stir in the melted butter, soya milk and maple syrup. Pour this into the bowl of flour, then add the remaining ingredients, and combine quickly without overworking (it's fine if there are a few lumps left in the mixture – you want it sticky rather than fluid). Spoon the mixture into the muffin tins.

Bake for 20–25 minutes until well risen and browned. Leave to cool in the tins for a few minutes before turning out, then allow to cool completely before serving or storing in an airtight tin.

Variation: if you like and you have the time, you can first plump up the dried fruit by soaking it in the juice from the orange, tossing from time to time, for about 30 minutes. This gives an even more moist result.

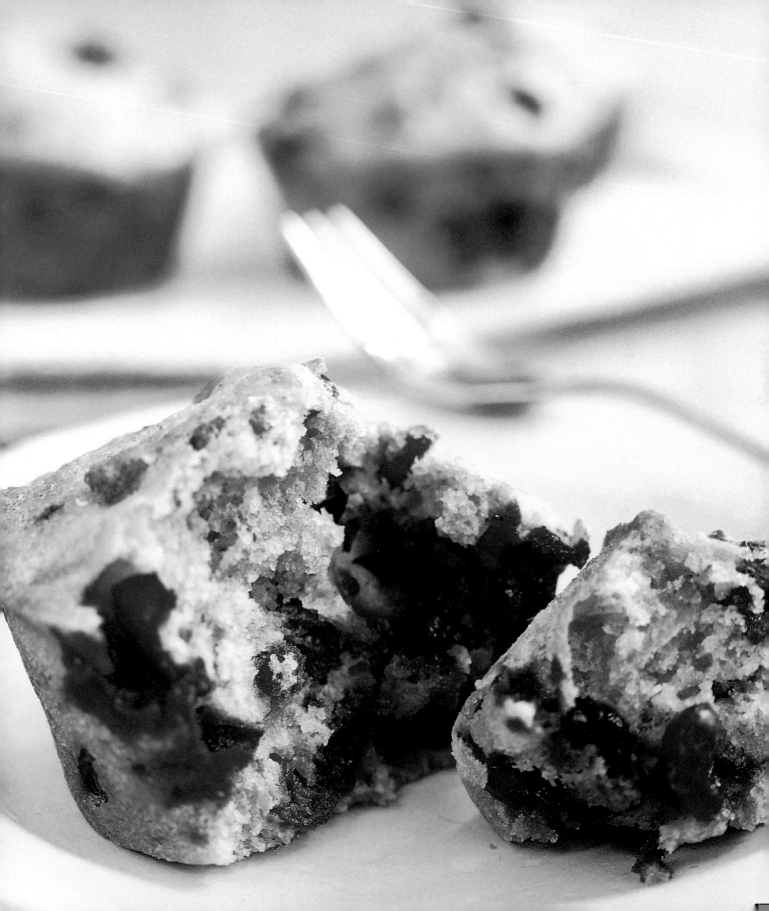

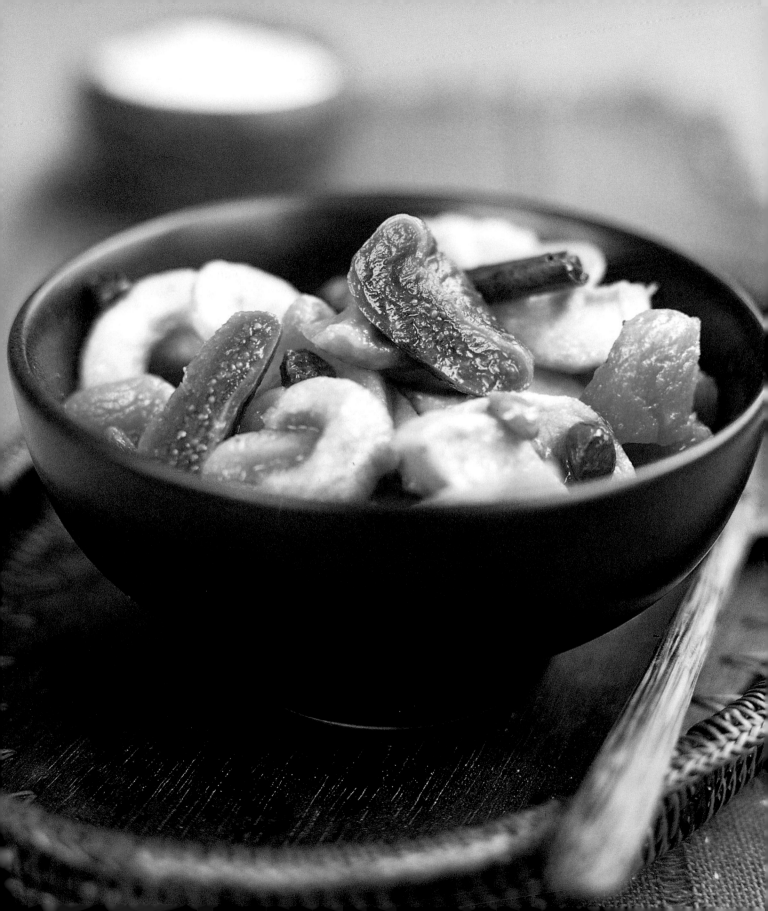

DRIED FRUIT COMPOTE WITH GINGERED FROMAGE FRAIS

P ★   E ★   A ★ ★ ★ ★

If you ever have a sugar craving, dried fruit is sweet as well as healthy. It is useful in alleviating constipation and contains high amounts of antioxidants. Dried figs are high in the soluble fibre pectin, which helps lower cholesterol levels. Both figs and apricots are rich in potassium, which helps with water retention. Lastly, ginger is good for the circulation. (See photograph opposite.)

SERVES 4–6
PREPARATION: 10 minutes
COOKING: 20 minutes, plus soaking

85 g/3 oz dried apple rings, halved
85 g/3 oz dried figs, cut into bite-sized pieces
85 g/3 oz dried apricots, cut into bite-sized pieces
40 g/1½ oz dried banana slices
40 g/1½ oz dried pineapple slices, broken up into pieces
40 g/1½ oz sultanas
150 ml/¼ pint dry cider
150 ml/¼ pint orange or apple juice
¼ cinnamon stick
1 tablespoon orange flower water, to serve

FOR THE GINGERED FROMAGE FRAIS:
Large chunk of fresh root ginger
2 tablespoons maple or date syrup, warmed
285 g/10 oz fromage frais

Put the dried fruit in a saucepan and pour over the cider and fruit juice. Drop in the cinnamon stick. Bring gently to just below boiling point, cover and simmer very gently for 15 minutes. Take off the heat and leave the fruit to soak and cool for at least 1 hour, ideally overnight.

To make the gingered fromage frais: press the root ginger through a garlic press and stir the resulting juice into the syrup. Stir that into the fromage frais.

Remove the cinnamon stick from the compôte (you can leave it in for presentation if you like, but do make sure no one crunches into it). Serve hot, warm or cold, sprinkled with the orange flower water and accompanied by the fromage frais.

Variation: instead of fromage frais you can use plain runny yoghurt, preferably soya yoghurt.

STRAWBERRY SMOOTHIE

P ★ ★ ★   E ★ ★   A ★ ★ ★ ★

This is a refreshing summer drink to set you up for the day. It delivers good amounts of phytoestrogens from the soya milk and antioxidants from the fruit. Strawberries contain more vitamin C than any other berry so they are good for the immune system and also help to produce collagen for skin and bone health.

MAKES about 550 ml/19 fl oz (2–3 good glasses)
PREPARATION: about 10 minutes

225 g/8 oz strawberries, sliced
225 ml/8 fl oz soya milk
1 tablespoon frozen orange juice concentrate, thawed
1 banana, chopped
Honey to taste (optional)

Put all the ingredients in a food processor with a handful of ice cubes and process until smooth. If necessary, sweeten to taste with a little honey.

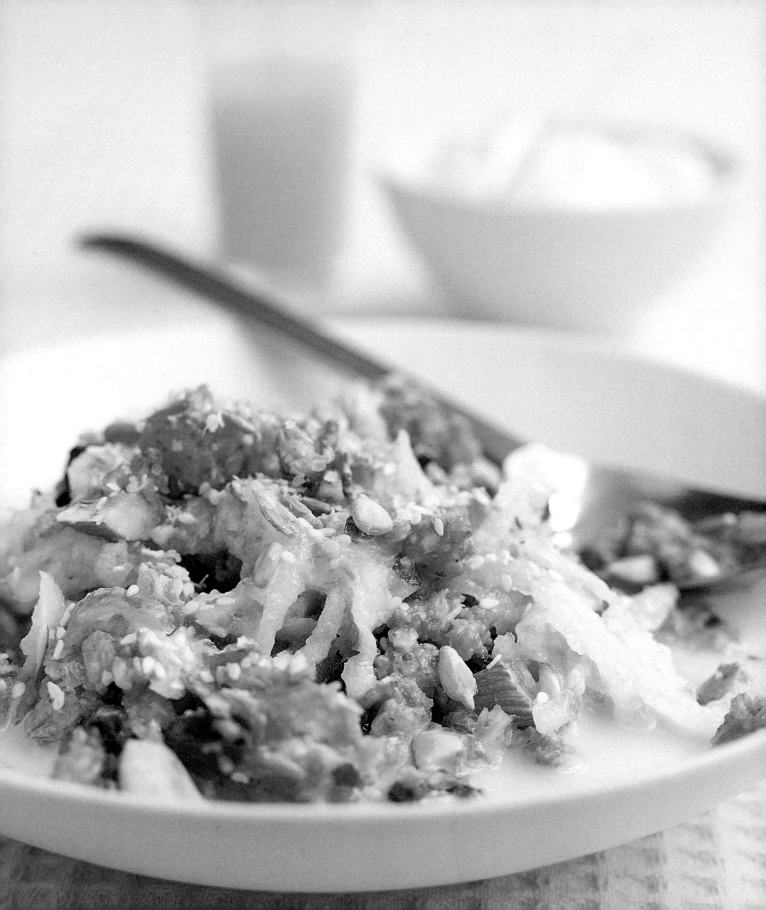

HOMEMADE LUXURY MUESLI

P ★★★★   E ★★★★★   A ★★★★★

It is wonderful to think that you can gain so many nutrients in just one breakfast. What's more, this luxury muesli (see photograph opposite) will set you up for the rest of the day and stop you from feeling peckish mid-morning.

The soya flour is full of phytoestrogens, as are the oats and barley. These last two are also excellent sources of fibre, noted for their ability to reduce heart disease. The seeds are also phytoestrogenic and, along with the nuts, supply essential fatty acids. The apricots are rich in the antioxidant beta-carotene and the oranges, apples and pears provide you with good amounts of vitamin C. Lastly, the live organic yoghurt is recommended for the digestive system as it contains beneficial bacteria.

SERVES 4
PREPARATION: 15 minutes, plus overnight soaking

4 tablespoons rolled oats
4 tablespoons barley kernels or flakes
55 g/2 oz soya flour
4 tablespoons raisins
55 g/2 oz dried apricots, chopped into chunks
2 large oranges
2 dessert apples
2 pears
Juice of 1 lemon
4 tablespoons good-quality runny honey or maple syrup
4 tablespoons unsalted mixed nuts, chopped
1 tablespoon linseeds
1 tablespoon sunflower seeds
1 tablespoon sesame seeds
Soya milk and organic live plain yoghurt, to serve

The night before, put the oats, barley, soya flour and dried fruit in a bowl. Pare the zest from 1 of the oranges and squeeze the juice of both. Add these to the bowl (along with any orange pulp that gathers in the grater) and toss well to mix. Leave to soak overnight.

In the morning, coarsely grate the unpeeled apples and pears on top of the soaked grains. Pour over the lemon juice. Add the honey or maple syrup and the chopped nuts, and mix well.

Finish by sprinkling with the linseeds, sunflower and sesame seeds. Serve with soya milk and some plain yoghurt.

POSH PORRIDGE

P ★★★★★   E ★★   A ★★★★

Oats, which make an excellent warming breakfast, are one of the best foods for keeping cholesterol under control as well as being phytoestrogenic. This particular porridge gives you that little extra boost to your health by using soya milk, soya cream and cinnamon – all sources of phytoestrogens.

The dried fruit is an excellent source of antioxidants as well as potassium, which helps with water retention. If you add a fruit purée made predominantly with berries you will be giving yourself extra antioxidants by way of their bioflavonoids. Bioflavonoids strengthen the collagen in the bone matrix, so helping to prevent osteoporosis.

SERVES 4
PREPARATION: about 5 minutes,
plus overnight soaking (if using coarse oatmeal)
COOKING: about 30 minutes for coarse oatmeal,
5–10 minutes for porridge or rolled oats,
plus a few minutes' cooling

55g/2oz oatmeal

450ml/¾ pint soya milk

100ml/3½ floz soya cream

3 tablespoons orange juice

1 teaspoon ground cinnamon

3 tablespoons maple syrup

55g/2oz seedless raisins

55g/2oz dried figs, chopped

55g/2oz dried apricots, chopped

Additional maple syrup, or a fresh fruit purée or fruit compôte (see page 79), to serve

If using coarse oatmeal, first soak it in water overnight.

Put the oatmeal (well drained if necessary) in a large heavy-based pan and add the soya milk. Bring to the boil, lower the heat and then simmer for 20–30 minutes for coarse oatmeal, or 3–4 minutes (check the packet's instructions) for porridge or rolled oats.

Remove from the pan from the heat and allow to cool slightly.

When cooler, stir in the soya cream, orange juice, cinnamon and maple syrup and mix well. Then stir in the dried fruit.

You can either serve the porridge warm or cold, topped with some more maple syrup or a fresh fruit purée, such as raspberry or strawberry, or dried fruit compôte (see page 79).

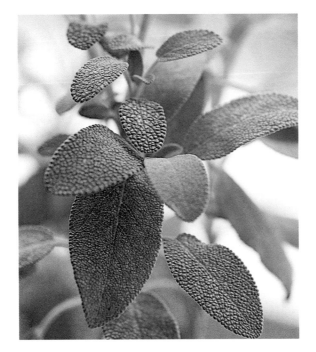

Lunches
and
light
meals

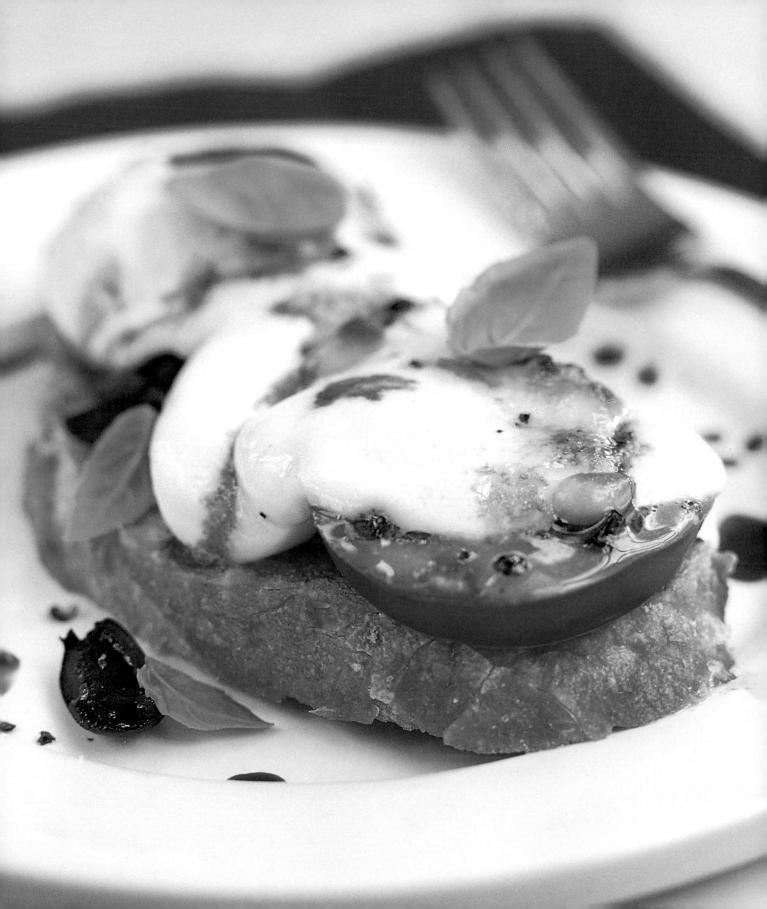

MOZZARELLA AND TOMATO GRATIN

P ★   E ★   A ★ ★ ★

Insalata tricolore remains an irresistible favourite for many food lovers; this dish (see photograph opposite) takes that wonderful combination of Mozzarella, tomato and basil and makes it even more tempting, by melting the cheese.

The tomatoes are an excellent source of lycopene, which may have a preventative effect against cancer, heart disease and degenerative eye conditions. The olives are valuable for their beneficial effects on the heart.

SERVES 4
PREPARATION: about 15 minutes
COOKING: about 5 minutes

350g/12oz vine-ripened tomatoes, sliced
Freshly ground sea salt and black pepper
Handful of basil, shredded, plus more sprigs to garnish
2 tablespoons pitted black olives, cut into slivers
2 tablespoons pine nuts
3 fresh (preferably buffalo) Mozzarella cheeses, each about 100g/3½oz, cut into slices
Balsamic vinegar

Preheat a hot grill. Arrange the tomato slices in the bottom of a medium-sized gratin dish and season well. Sprinkle over the shredded basil, olive slivers and half the pine nuts.

Arrange the cheese slices over the top and sprinkle over the remaining pine nuts and a few drops of balsamic vinegar here and there. Season again with pepper.

Grill until the Mozzarella is nicely melted and the bottom of the dish is good and hot.

Serve at once, garnished with the reserved sprigs of basil.

Variation: for a more substantial dish, try adding some rinsed and drained anchovy fillets to the layer between the tomatoes and the cheese. They add a more sophisticated flavour. The gratin is also delicious served on thick slices of ciabatta bread instead of in the dish, to make crostini.

COURGETTE RISOTTO

P ★ ★ ★   E ★   A ★ ★ ★

This risotto sounds deceptively plain, but make it with really fresh firm young courgettes and you will enjoy both the vegetable and risotto in a way you haven't been able to appreciate either before.

The miso broth gives you a good amount of phytoestrogens and the courgettes are an excellent source of beta-carotene, vitamin C and folic acid. Beta-carotene is a powerful antioxidant, effective in delaying ageing and preventing cancer. It may come as a surprise, but just a small portion of courgettes (100g/3½oz) provides you with more than a quarter of your daily needs of vitamin C – which is the same as one serving of this delicious creamy dish.

Nowadays arborio is probably the most common of the Italian *superfino* rice varieties offered as a risotto rice, but when you get the chance do try carnarole, Roma or vialone nano as an alternative.

SERVES 4
PREPARATION: about 5 minutes
COOKING: 35–40 minutes

*1.75 litres/3¼ pints miso broth (see page 176)
or good-quality vegetable stock (see page 177)*

85g/3oz butter

2 tablespoons olive oil

1 onion, diced

350g/12oz risotto rice (see above)

4 tablespoons dry white wine (optional)

Freshly ground sea salt and black pepper

450g/1lb courgettes, sliced at an angle and not too thinly

55g/2oz grated Parmesan cheese

Heat the miso broth or stock, and when it is almost boiling turn the heat down and keep it at a very gentle simmer.

Heat half the butter with the oil in a heavy-based pan and fry the onion until translucent. Add the rice and stir for a minute or two until every grain is coated and shiny with oil and butter. Add the wine if using and allow to boil off, stirring. Then add the stock a ladleful at a time, stirring it in and not adding the next ladleful until it is well absorbed.

After about 10 minutes, season and add the courgettes. Continue adding the stock and stirring. Taste after 20 minutes. The rice should still have a discernible bite and the texture of the risotto should be thick and porridge-like. If you find you have used up all the stock but the rice is not quite done, finish with ladlefuls of boiling water.

Remove the risotto from the heat, stir in the remaining butter and the cheese, cover and leave to stand for 3 minutes. Serve immediately.

Variation: make this into a special-occasion dish by adding a good pinch of saffron strands to the stock and adding some shredded basil leaves at the end with the butter and cheese.

PASTA WITH CRUSHED NUT VINAIGRETTE

P ★★★   E ★★★   A ★

The interesting nutty flavour that infuses this pasta belies its simplicity. From the linseeds and wholemeal pasta you will get phytoestrogens, plus gain benefits for your heart from the olive oil. Walnuts are rich in essential fatty acids and so are especially good for the heart and joints.

SERVES 4

PREPARATION: about 10 minutes

COOKING: about 15 minutes, depending on the pasta

Freshly ground sea salt and black pepper

450g/1lb (preferably wholemeal) pasta shapes, such as shells or spirals

50g/2oz grated Parmesan cheese, to serve

FOR THE CRUSHED NUT VINAIGRETTE:

2 tablespoons extra-virgin olive oil

1 tablespoon linseed oil

2 teaspoons balsamic vinegar

85g/3oz shelled walnuts, coarsely chopped or crushed

Put about 4.5 litres/8 pints of water in a large pan and bring to the boil. Salt and add the pasta. Cook, stirring occasionally, until the pasta is *al dente*, ie soft but still offering some resistance when you bite it.

While the pasta is cooking, make the vinaigrette: whisk all the ingredients together well (or shake to an emulsion in a sealed jar), reserving about a tablespoon of the chopped nuts for garnish and adding seasoning to taste.

Drain the pasta well, pour over the vinaigrette and toss to coat well. Serve immediately, garnished with the reserved nuts and some Parmesan, with the rest of the grated cheese served in a bowl.

PASTA WITH BROCCOLI AND ANCHOVIES

P ★★   E ★★★   A ★

Anchovies are an excellent source of Omega 3 essential fatty acids, which are good for the heart and the skin and joints. The wholemeal pasta provides the necessary phytoestrogens and the broccoli helps to guard against cancer.

SERVES 4
PREPARATION: about 10 minutes
COOKING: about 15 minutes, depending on the pasta

Freshly ground sea salt and black pepper
450g/1lb (preferably wholemeal) pasta noodles, such as tagliatelle
450g/1lb broccoli, cut into bite-sized pieces
3 tablespoons olive oil
6 garlic cloves, thinly sliced
4–6 anchovy fillets, rinsed, drained and chopped
Grated Parmesan cheese, to serve

Cook the pasta as described in the previous recipe. While the pasta is cooking, bring a large pan of salted water to the boil. Blanch the broccoli in the boiling water for 1 minute only after it comes back to the boil. Drain, refresh in cold water to stop it cooking any more and drain well.

Heat the oil in a large frying pan until almost hot and add the garlic. Sauté until just turning golden-brown in colour. Add the broccoli and anchovies with seasoning and sauté for a minute or two more.

Drain the cooked pasta well and either return to the pan or put in a large warmed serving bowl. Pour over the contents of the frying pan, adding more seasoning if necessary, and toss well. Serve accompanied by the cheese.

PASTA WITH FRIED SAGE LEAVES

P ★★★   E ★★   A ★

This is another simple but fresh-tasting pasta dish which uses an excellent herb for the menopause, sage. Sage is known to help reduce hot flushes and, together with the phytoestrogens in the wholemeal pasta, makes for a healthy combination. (See photograph, page 21.)

SERVES 4
PREPARATION: about 10 minutes
COOKING: about 15 minutes, depending on the pasta

Freshly ground sea salt and black pepper
450g/1lb (preferably wholemeal) pasta noodles, such as tagliatelle
2 tablespoons olive oil
25g/1oz butter
Large handful of sage
55g/2oz pine nuts
55g/2oz grated Parmesan cheese, plus more to serve

Cook the pasta as for the Pasta with Crushed Nut Vinaigrette (see opposite page).

While the pasta is cooking, heat the oil and butter in a large frying pan and fry half the sage leaves on both sides until crisp. Remove from the pan with tongs and drain on a layer of kitchen paper. Add the pine nuts to the pan and sauté until golden. Finely chop the remaining sage and stir into the pine nuts.

Drain the cooked pasta well and either return to the pan or put in a large warmed serving bowl. Pour over the contents of the frying pan, add the Parmesan and seasoning to taste.

Toss with the whole sage leaves to serve, accompanied by more grated cheese.

Refried Bean Tortillas with Tomato Salsa

P ★ ★ ★ ★ ★   E ★   A ★ ★ ★ ★ ★

Wonderfully, refried bean tortillas are packed with phytoestrogens from the beans, miso, garlic and corn. The tomatoes in the salsa supply a good level of antioxidants, which are also found in the red pepper.

Onions are known to help prevent osteoporosis and the garlic is reported to have anti-cancer effects. The limes are an excellent source of vitamin C, which helps to combat free radicals and prevent premature ageing.

This dish makes excellent party food if you cut the tortillas into small bite-sized wedges and spread the beans on them. Either way, it is delicious served with guacamole (see page 58).

SERVES 4

PREPARATION: about 20 minutes

COOKING: about 20 minutes, plus cooking beans if not using canned

6 tablespoons olive oil

450g/1lb cooked (or tinned) pinto beans or red kidney beans

Freshly ground sea salt and black pepper

3–4 tablespoons hot miso broth (see page 176)

4–6 spring onions, chopped

115g/4oz Cheddar cheese, grated

8 corn tortillas or 4 flour tortillas

1 Cos lettuce heart, shredded

FOR THE TOMATO SALSA:

6 large ripe but firm tomatoes, preferably plum or vine

1 red onion, diced

1 garlic clove, very finely chopped

1 large red pepper, deseeded and diced

1–2 red chilli(es), deseeded and chopped

Juice of 2 limes

Large handful of coriander, chopped, plus some whole leaves to garnish

Freshly ground sea salt and black pepper

First make the salsa: halve the tomatoes, scoop out the seeds and discard them. Dice the flesh (skin included) and put it in a serving bowl, together with the red onion, garlic, pepper, chilli, lime juice, chopped coriander and seasoning. Mix well, cover and chill while you fry the beans.

Heat half the oil in a large frying pan and add the beans (you will need to drain them if they are tinned). Season and, if they are very dry, add a few spoonfuls of the hot miso broth. Fry the beans briskly, stirring frequently with a wooden spoon. As the beans soften, start to press them down with the spoon to form a large cake and keep cooking until the cake is glazed and will move as one piece in the pan.

Move this to one side of the pan and turn it over like a pancake, then cook the other side in the same way. Turn off the heat under the pan and sprinkle the beans with the spring onions followed by the cheese. Cover.

At the same time, cook the tortillas: heat the remaining oil in a frying pan and, when it is hot, dip each of the tortillas into it, one at a time, for about 15 seconds each.

Once the cheese has melted, serve the refried beans on a bed of shredded lettuce with the tortillas (break flour tortillas into pieces) and the salsa in separate bowls.

Variation: for an even more substantial and phyto-packed version of this dish, sprinkle some bite-sized pieces of cooked broccoli on top of the beans with the spring onions.

CRAB ENCHILADAS

P ★ ★ ★   E ★   A ★ ★ ★ ★

If you are aware that spicy food can bring on a hot flush then omit the chilli from this recipe. Chilli, like mustard and garlic, in fact has the ability to shift excess mucus, which can be welcome. The miso gives the dish a rich flavour and is a source of phytoestrogens, as is the excellent vegetable, celery. Celery contains potassium which helps alleviate water retention, often a source of weight gain at the menopause. Celery also has anti-inflammatory properties.

Crab not only lends a delicate flavour to any dish but is also an excellent source of several nutrients. These include the vitamins B2 and B5, good amounts of magnesium and zinc – both vital for your bones – and potassium, which is beneficial for water retention. The tomatoes are rich in the antioxidant lycopene. Parsley is a source of calcium, vitamins A and C and also iron and potassium, making it a good diuretic. Corn, a traditional grain used in many cultures, is likewise a good source of potassium and iron.

SERVES 4
PREPARATION: about 25 minutes
COOKING: about 20 minutes

200g/7oz dressed fresh crab meat (brown and white)
Juice of 1 lime
2 tablespoons chopped coriander, plus some whole leaves to garnish
1 celery stalk, finely chopped
½ small bulb of fennel, with fronds, finely chopped
Dash of no-added-sugar Worcestershire sauce
About 3 tablespoons olive oil, plus more for greasing
8 corn tortillas
200g/7oz Mozzarella cheese, shredded

FOR THE CHILLI TOMATO SAUCE:
2 tablespoons olive oil
1 large onion, diced
1 garlic clove, finely chopped
1–2 hot red chilli(es), deseeded and finely chopped
100ml/3½ fl oz red wine (optional)
400g/14oz tinned chopped plum tomatoes
3 tablespoons tomato paste
1 tablespoon parsley, chopped
1–2 teaspoons miso dissolved in 300ml/½ pint boiling water
Freshly ground sea salt and black pepper

First make the chilli tomato sauce: heat the oil in a heavy-based pan and sauté the onion in it gently until just translucent, then add the garlic and chilli, and sauté for about 1 minute more. Add the wine if using and boil rapidly to reduce it to a sticky liquid. Stir in the tomatoes with their liquid, the tomato paste, parsley and miso solution. Mix well, season and simmer for about 30 minutes, until it has a good thick sauce-like consistency.

Preheat the oven to 200°C/400°F/Gas 6.

To make the filling, mix the crab meat, lime juice, coriander, celery, fennel and Worcestershire sauce into half of the chilli tomato sauce. Adjust the seasoning to taste.

Heat the oil in a frying pan and dip each of the tortillas into it, one at a time, for about 15 seconds on each side. This will make them pliable. Place some filling in the centre of each and roll the tortilla around this loosely. Place in a lightly oiled ovenproof dish big enough to hold all the enchiladas in a single layer.

Once they are all arranged in the dish, adjust the seasoning of the remaining tomato sauce and pour this over them (each enchilada should be almost covered). Sprinkle with the cheese and bake for about 15 minutes, until bubbling.

Serve garnished with whole coriander leaves.

Tofu Vegetable Quiche

P ★★★★   E ★★   A ★★

This quiche is an unusual way to serve tofu and makes an interesting change. It is full of healthy ingredients, including the tofu, tahini and broccoli, which all deliver phytoestrogens. Made from sesame seeds, the tahini is also a rich source of calcium. Health food shops should sell pre-baked savoury tart shells; otherwise use an ordinary pastry tart suitable for quiche, but make sure it is made with wholemeal flour.

SERVES 4
PREPARATION: about 15 minutes
COOKING: 25–30 minutes

2 tablespoons tahini

3 tablespoons soy sauce

900 g/2 lb soft tofu, mashed

1 tablespoon arrowroot

450 g/1 lb broccoli, cut into small bite-sized pieces

1 pre-baked savoury tart shell

Preheat the oven to 150°C/300°F/Gas 2.

Combine the tahini, soy sauce and the tofu in a bowl. Dissolve the arrowroot in 75 ml/2 fl oz water and combine with the tahini mixture in a saucepan. Bring to a simmer and continue to cook over a moderate heat for 7–10 minutes.

Meanwhile, in a separate pan, steam the broccoli pieces until they are just beginning to get tender. Add the broccoli to the tofu mixture and spoon into the pie shell. Bake in the preheated oven for 8 minutes.

Herring with Oatmeal

P ★★   E ★★★★   A ★

Herrings (see photograph opposite) are rich in Omega 3 oils. The oatmeal is not only a phyto-estrogen but also a good source of fibre, and the oat bran (in the oats) beneficial for the heart.

SERVES 4
PREPARATION: about 10 minutes
COOKING: about 25 minutes

4 boned herrings

1 egg

Freshly ground sea salt and black pepper

About 100 g/3½ oz fine oatmeal or rolled oats

2 tablespoons olive oil

About 15 g/½ oz butter

1 tablespoon chopped parsley, to garnish

Lemon wedges, to serve

If you can't get your fishmonger to bone the herring for you then cut off the heads of the fish and gut them, cutting them open from head to tail. Run your thumbs down the back to detach the spines, then ease these away from the skin and flesh. Use tweezers to pull out as many of the remaining bones as possible.

In a large shallow bowl, beat the egg with some salt and pepper. Put the oatmeal in another bowl and season that.

Heat the oil and butter in a large frying pan. Dip each flattened fish first in the egg, making sure it is coated well, and then in the oatmeal, pressing firmly. Fry over a moderate heat for about 6 minutes on each side. You'll probably have to do this in batches, so layer the cooked herrings on paper towels and keep warm in a low oven while you cook the rest.

Serve garnished with parsley and lemon wedges.

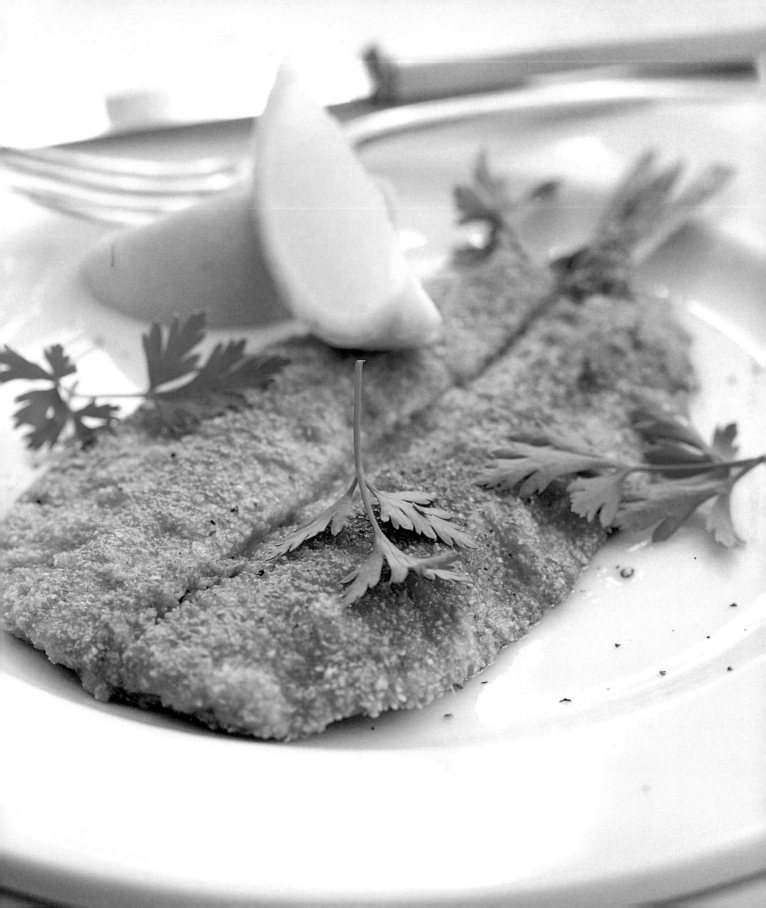

GRILLED SARDINES WITH FENNEL AND PINE NUTS

P ★★   E ★★★★   A ★

What a delicious mix of ingredients there are in this dish, and how good they are for you! The sardines and pine nuts supply both Omega 3 and Omega 6 essential fatty acids – so beneficial for the skin and joints – and there are phytoestrogens present in both the fennel and the parsley.

Nutty mash (see page 112) makes an excellent accompaniment to these beautifully aromatic sardines.

SERVES 4

PREPARATION: about 20 minutes, plus at least 1 hour's marinating

COOKING: about 10–15 minutes

About 900g/2lb fresh sardines, scaled and gutted

55g/2oz pine nuts

Lemon wedges, to serve

FOR THE MARINADE:

150ml/¼ pint olive oil

Juice of 1 lemon

Juice of 1 small orange

2–3 garlic cloves, crushed

½ fennel bulb, cut into matchstick strips, any feathery fronds reserved to garnish

2 tablespoons chopped parsley, plus more whole sprigs to garnish

Freshly ground sea salt and black pepper

At least an hour ahead, make the marinade by mixing all the ingredients and seasoning well. Transfer to a shallow bowl and add the sardines.

Leave to marinate in a cool place, turning from time to time.

Preheat a hot grill or barbecue, or a griddle pan.

Shaking as much of the marinade off as you can and, reserving it, grill the sardines for about 5–8 minutes on each side, depending on size, until well coloured and cooked through.

While they are cooking, put the marinade in a small pan and bring to a simmer. Simmer for 4–5 minutes, until the fennel is just tender. At the same time, roast the pine nuts in a dry frying pan until lightly browned and aromatic.

Serve the grilled sardines with the marinade spooned over them and the pine nuts sprinkled on top of that. Garnish with any reserved fennel fronds and parsley sprigs, and serve with lemon wedges.

GADO GADO SALAD

P ★★★★   E ★★★   A ★★★★★

Indonesian gado gado (see photograph opposite) is an unusual combination of hot and cold ingredients, with a hot peanut sauce poured over a crunchy salad. Not only is this lunch tasty, it also has excellent health-giving ingredients.

Although we don't want to eat a lot of fried food, the occasional fried tofu, etc is fine as long as it is balanced with other ingredients. The tofu is very high in phytoestrogens and so are the beansprouts. Cauliflower is one of the cruciferous vegetables known for their anti-cancer properties as well as their excellent vitamin C content. Watercress is both an excellent source of vitamin C and beta-carotene, and the carrots likewise. Cucumbers are an interesting vegetable in that they contain specific bioflavonoids which can prevent the cell-binding activity of certain cancer-causing hormones.

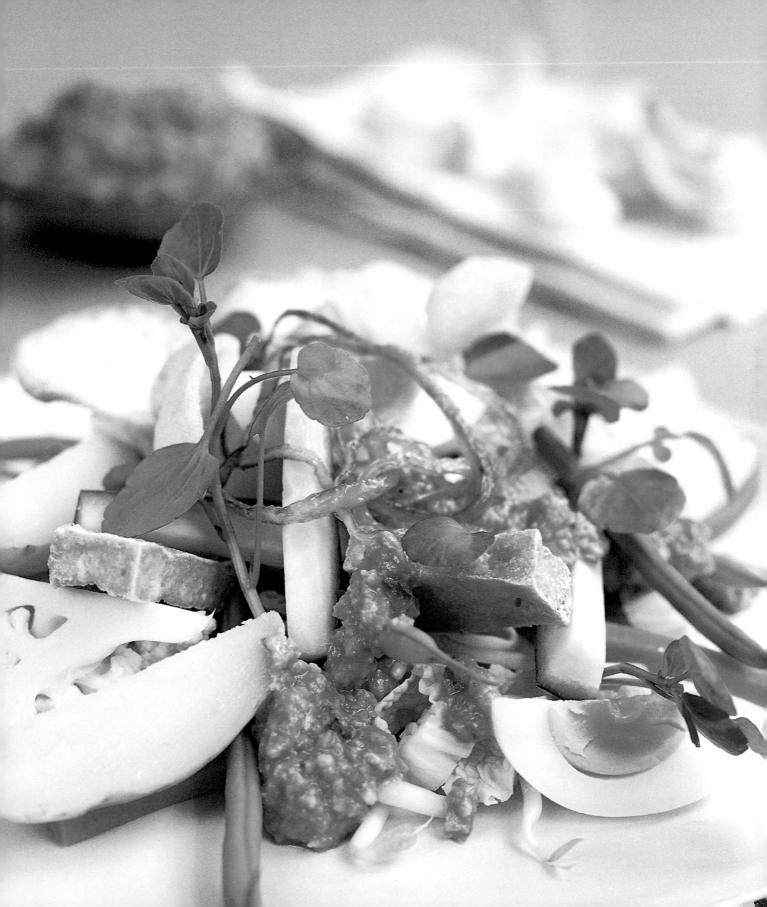

SERVES 4–6

PREPARATION: about 25 minutes

COOKING: about 15 minutes (for the potatoes, eggs and onions), plus making the sauce

About 450 ml/¾ pint peanut sauce (see page 182), reheated if necessary

200 g/7 oz tofu, cut into 1-cm/½-in slices

1 tablespoon olive oil

FOR THE SALAD:

4–6 carrots, cut into matchstick strips

175 g/6 oz beansprouts

175 g/6 oz fine green beans

115 g/4 oz cauliflower florets

1 tablespoon linseeds

1 small head of Chinese leaves, thinly sliced

FOR THE GARNISH:

½ cucumber, cut into thickish matchstick strips

4 hard-boiled eggs, cut into wedges

4 cooked potatoes, cut into wedges

Large handful of watercress or baby spinach

1 large onion, sliced and dry-fried until crisp

Large handful of no-added-sugar prawn crackers

First make the peanut sauce (see page 182). Keep warm. Then sauté the tofu in a little olive oil, until it is crunchy.

Combine this and all the other salad ingredients (you can either serve this dish in individual portions or in one big bowl). Pour the warm peanut sauce over the salad, then arrange the garnish ingredients: place the cucumber, egg and potato around the edge and pile the watercress or spinach and dry-fried onions in the centre.

Serve immediately, sprinkled with the no-added-sugar prawn crackers.

PASTA SALAD PRIMAVERA

P ★★★   E ★★★   A ★★★

All the spring vegetables in this pasta combine to offer good phytoestrogens, especially the carrots, peas, green beans and the parsley. The tomatoes and courgettes supply plenty of antioxidants and the essential oils are covered by the linseed oil. (See photograph opposite.)

SERVES 4

PREPARATION: about 20 minutes

COOKING: about 15 minutes, plus cooling

Freshly ground sea salt and black pepper

225 g/8 oz (preferably wholemeal) pasta shapes, such as penne, spirals, bows or shells, or a mixture

6 baby carrots, whole or halved lengthwise if thick

115 g/4 oz fine green beans

6 baby courgettes, halved lengthwise

15 g/½ oz butter

115 g/4 oz mange-tout peas, cut into strips if large

4 spring onions, quartered at an angle

115/4 oz cherry tomatoes (preferably Santa baby plum tomatoes), halved

55 g/2 oz pitted whole black olives

55 g/2 oz Parmesan cheese

FOR THE PARSLEY VINAIGRETTE:

3 tablespoons olive oil

2 tablespoons linseed oil

1 tablespoon balsamic vinegar

1 tablespoon fresh parsley, chopped

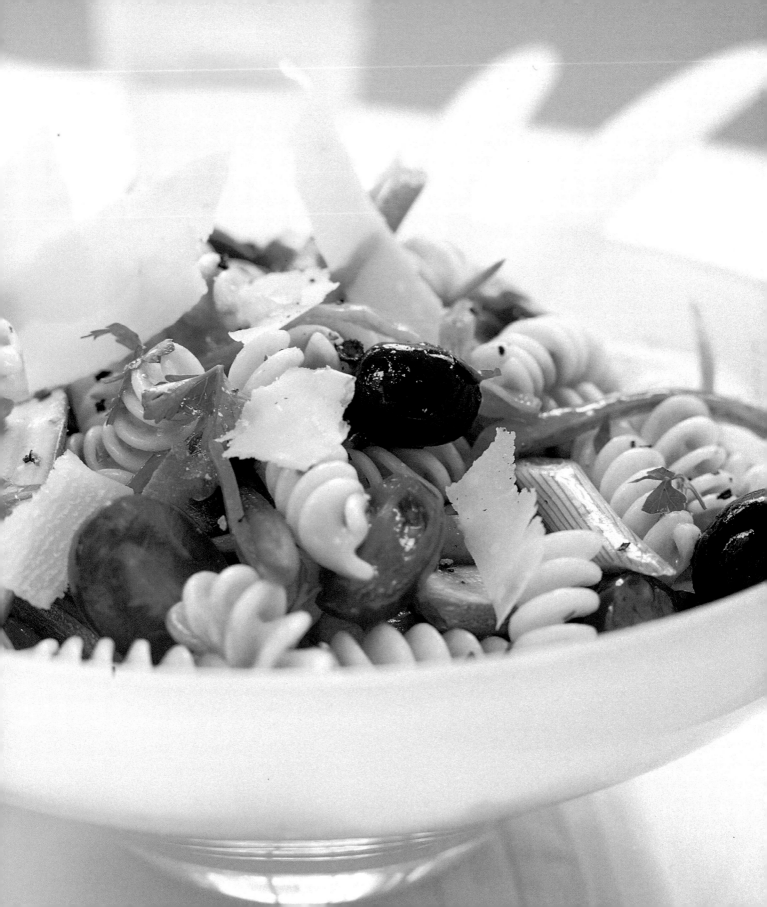

Cook the pasta as for the Pasta with Crushed Nut Vinaigrette (see page 86).

While the pasta is cooking, make the vinaigrette: whisk all the ingredients together well (or shake to an emulsion in a sealed jar), adding seasoning to taste.

Drain the cooked pasta well, pour over half the vinaigrette and toss well to coat thoroughly, then leave to cool.

Meanwhile, prepare the vegetables: in separate small pans of boiling salted water cook the carrots, beans and courgettes until just tender. As they are done, drain, refresh in cold water and drain again.

Melt the butter in a frying pan over low-to-moderate heat and sauté the mange-tout and spring onions until just beginning to wilt. Add all the remaining vegetables and toss to coat.

Transfer to a serving bowl, add half the olives and the remaining vinaigrette and toss to coat, then mix in the pasta. Dot with the remaining olives and with long shavings of the Parmesan made using a swivel peeler.

RUSSIAN SALAD DELUXE WITH TOFU DRESSING

P ★★★★★   E ★★★★   A ★★★★★

This salad is truly deluxe as it has such an interesting variety of vegetables. It delivers a superb mix of phytoestrogens in the form of tofu, fennel, carrots, peas and apples. The essential fatty acid content is also high, from the linseed oil and the walnuts. And lastly, the mix of colours provided by the green peas, orange carrots, red beetroots, black and green grapes and the apples gives plenty of different and important antioxidants.

SERVES 4

PREPARATION: about 25 minutes

COOKING: about 15–20 minutes, plus cooling

85g/3oz waxy potatoes, peeled

85g/3oz baby carrots, scrubbed

85g/3oz peas

85g/3oz cooked beetroots, peeled

½ fennel bulb, cored and finely chopped, fronds reserved to garnish

85g/3oz grapes (black and green), halved and deseeded

2 large eating apples, cored and diced (leave skin on)

85g/3oz walnuts

50g/2oz capers

Little Gem lettuces, shredded, to serve

FOR THE TOFU DRESSING:

250g/9oz tofu

3 tablespoons cider vinegar

2 tablespoons olive oil

1 tablespoon linseed oil

1 tablespoon soy sauce

Freshly ground sea salt and black pepper

Cook the potatoes, carrots and peas in separate pans of boiling salted water until just tender. Drain well and, when cool, cut the potatoes and carrots into 1-cm/½-in cubes. Cut the beetroots into the same sized cubes.

Put all these in a large, preferably glass, salad bowl together with the fennel, grapes (reserving a few of each colour for garnish), apples, walnuts and capers. Toss lightly to mix.

Make the dressing: blend all the ingredients in a food processor until smooth. Season to taste. Spoon over the salad and toss so that all the ingredients are lightly coated but are still identifiable.

Serve on beds of shredded lettuce, garnished with fennel fronds and more grape halves.

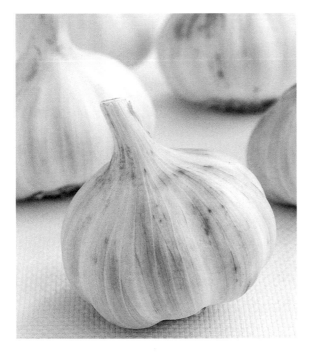

*Family
and
weekday
fare*

VEGETABLE YOGHURT MOUSSAKA

P ★★★★ E ★★ A ★★★★

Made with added nuts and dried fruit, this moussaka is the perfect thing for casual entertaining, and if you use all or part wild mushrooms, you have quite a sophisticated dish.

The moussaka contains phytoestrogens in the form of the soya flour, soya yoghurt, soya milk and mushrooms. The almonds give good amounts of essential fatty acids, and antioxidants are provided by the tomatoes, apricots and courgettes – which are also an excellent source of beta-carotene, vitamin C and folic acid.

I have always suspected there was a better way of preparing aubergines than all that business with salting and then frying them in, ultimately, gallons of oil. I discovered this idea of first baking them in a spicy coating in the wonderful *American New Basics Cookbook* by the Silver Palate people. It produces a much lighter and tastier result.

SERVES 6–8
PREPARATION: about 40 minutes
COOKING: about 1¼ hours

About 4 tablespoons olive oil, plus more for greasing
1 tablespoon ground cumin
1 tablespoon ground ginger
1 tablespoon ground cinnamon
2 teaspoons freshly grated nutmeg
85 g/3 oz soya flour
Freshly ground sea salt and black pepper
100 ml/3½ fl oz soya milk
900 g/2 lb large aubergines, thinly sliced
2 recipe quantities basic tomato sauce (see page 178)
450 g/1 lb courgettes, sliced
225 g/8 oz chestnut mushrooms, sliced
25 g/1 oz butter
85 g/3 oz split almonds, lightly toasted (optional)
85 g/3 oz dried apricots, chopped (optional)
85 g/3 oz seedless raisins (optional)
2 eggs, lightly beaten
450 ml/¾ pint plain runny yoghurt, ideally soya yoghurt
2 tablespoons lemon juice
2 tablespoons fresh mint, chopped
55 g/2 oz Parmesan cheese, freshly grated

Preheat the oven to 190°C/375°F/Gas 5 and oil a baking sheet and a large ovenproof casserole.

In a shallow bowl, mix half the spices with the flour and 1 teaspoon each of salt and pepper. Put the milk in another shallow bowl. One by one, dip the aubergine slices in the soya milk and then in the seasoned flour, shaking off any excess, and arrange on a baking sheet. Bake for 25 minutes only.

While they are baking, make the tomato sauce, adding the remaining spices to the tomatoes. In separate pans or one after the other, lightly sauté the courgettes and mushrooms in the butter with the oil until just softened. Season to taste and set aside in a warm place.

When the aubergine slices are ready, remove them from the oven and reduce the setting to 170°C/350°F/Gas 4. Put a layer of one-quarter of the aubergines in the bottom of the casserole. If you are using them, mix the almonds and dried fruit into the tomato sauce when it is ready.

Spoon one-third of the sauce over the aubergine layer, followed by the mushrooms, then another layer of sauce, a layer of courgettes, a final layer of tomato sauce and a final top layer of aubergine.

In a bowl, mix the eggs into the yoghurt, followed by the lemon juice and mint. Pour over the dish. Sprinkle the Parmesan over the top and bake for 45 minutes, until uniformly golden brown.

VEGETABLE CHILLI

P ★★★★   E ★★★   A ★★★★

Chilli is another ever-popular family meal, wholesome and spicy. This dish includes phytoestrogens from the kidney beans, miso broth and carrots; excellent helpings of antioxidants from the carrots, courgettes and tomatoes; and essential fatty acids from the linseeds if you choose to add them before serving. Plenty of essential nutrients are also supplied by the seaweed flakes, including iodine for a healthy working thyroid.

If hot food tends to bring on hot flushes, you would do better to omit the chilli and enjoy this dish for its wonderful vegetables and herbs.

SERVES 4–6
PREPARATION: about 30 minutes
COOKING: about 1 hour

4 tablespoons olive oil

1 teaspoon ground cumin

1 teaspoon ground cinnamon

1 teaspoon fennel seeds

2 teaspoons sesame seeds

1 teaspoon dried oregano

Chilli powder to taste (optional)

2 onions, chopped

2 garlic cloves, finely chopped

2 peppers, preferably of different colours, deseeded and cut into thick strips

2 hot red chillies, deseeded (if you don't want the dish too hot) and finely chopped

4 tablespoons red wine (optional)

3–4 carrots, cut into batons

3–4 courgettes, cut into batons

400g/14oz tinned chopped plum tomatoes

3 tablespoons tomato paste

About 850ml/1½ pints miso broth (see page 176) or fish or shellfish stock (see page 177)

2 large tins of red kidney beans, drained

Handful of mixed seaweed flakes

Freshly ground sea salt and black pepper

3 tablespoons chopped coriander, plus more sprigs to garnish

Juice of 1 lemon

TO SERVE:

Sour cream

Red onion, chopped

Mature Cheddar cheese, grated

Heat the oil in a large and deep heavy-based pan. When hot, cook all the spices, seeds and oregano in the oil for a minute or two over a moderate heat, until aromatic. Then lower the heat and sauté the onion until translucent. Add the garlic, pepper strips and chillies, and sauté briefly until just beginning to soften. Add the red wine (if using) and cook, uncovered, until reduced right down.

At the same time, in a separate pan sauté the carrot batons in the remaining oil for about 5 minutes. Then add the courgettes and sauté together for about 5 minutes more, until both vegetables are just softened.

When the wine has reduced, add the tomatoes, tomato paste and stock to the pan with the beans, sautéed vegetables and seaweed. Season to taste and bring to the boil. Lower the heat, cover and simmer gently for about 30 minutes.

Stir in the coriander and lemon juice and cook for 10 minutes more. Serve with separate bowls of sour cream, chopped red onion and grated Cheddar.

Variation: if you want to boost the dish's phyto content, stir a spoonful or two of linseeds into the chilli just before serving or mix into the sour cream.

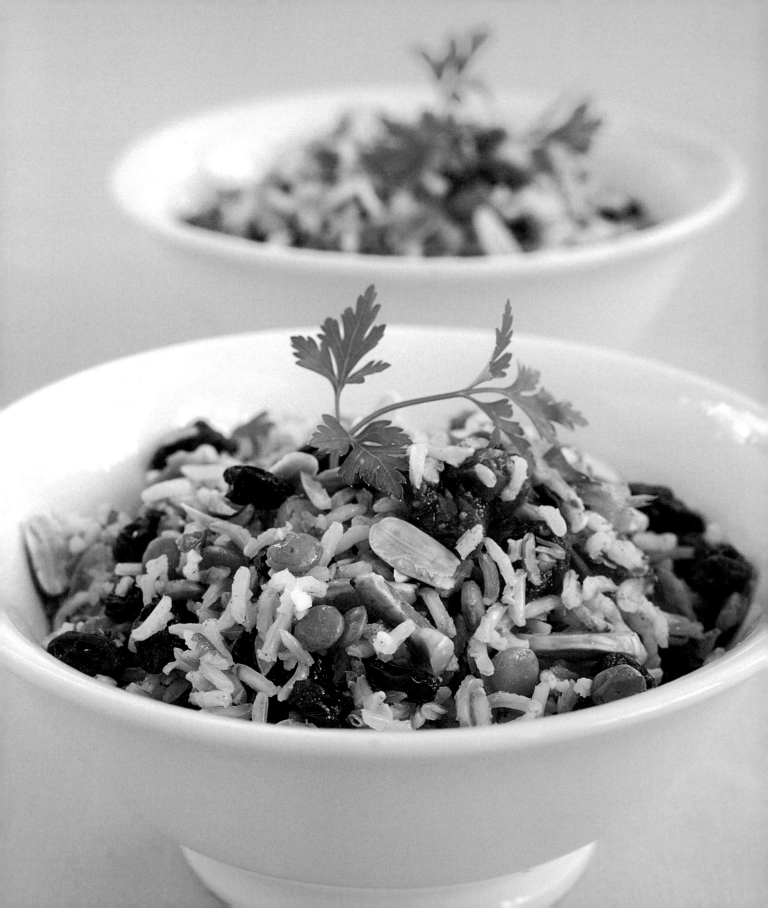

LENTIL AND FRUIT PILAF

P ★★★★★   E ★★   A ★★

Lentils are a wonderful source of phytoestrogens because they contain all four isoflavones. Further plant hormones are found in the rice, cinnamon, parsley and soya yoghurt.

Using the almonds only very lightly toasted or raw will give a good amount of essential oils, and the dried fruits are rich in antioxidants. (See photograph opposite.)

SERVES 4
PREPARATION: about 15 minutes
COOKING: about 50 minutes

175 g/6 oz green lentils
Freshly ground sea salt and black pepper
450 g/1 lb basmati rice
125 g/4½ oz seedless raisins
2–3 pitted dates, chopped
2–3 dried figs, chopped
1 tablespoon rose water or orange flower water
1 teaspoon ground cinnamon
2 tablespoons chopped flat-leaved parsley, plus more whole sprigs to garnish
125 g/4½ oz split blanched almonds, lightly toasted in a dry frying pan
3 tablespoons extra-virgin olive oil
Yoghurt, preferably soya yoghurt, to serve

Rinse the lentils well and put them in a large pan of fresh water. Bring to the boil and boil for 20–30 minutes until just tender, adding salt only after the lentils start to soften (otherwise the skins toughen). Drain well.

While the lentils are cooking, rinse the rice well under running cold water, drain and then put into a pan of boiling salted water. Bring back to the boil, stir well, lower the heat and simmer until just tender, 8–10 minutes. Drain well.

Mix the dried fruit, rose water or orange flower water and cinnamon in a bowl.

In a large heavy-based pan, arrange layers of rice, lentils and dried fruit, seasoning each layer and sprinkling some parsley and almonds over the top (reserving some of each for garnish). Drizzle over the olive oil, cover and cook very gently for 15–20 minutes.

Serve garnished with some parsley sprigs and accompanied by a bowl of yoghurt.

SIMPLE PAELLA

P ★★★   E ★★★★   A ★★★★

Paella is the perfect family meal: full of goodness, colour and flavour and easy to prepare. The miso broth, fennel, garlic and peppers supply the plant hormones.

The mussels, as well as being a good source of essential fatty acids, also provide the B vitamins and are rich in selenium, iron and iodine. Iodine, from natural sources, is particularly useful at the menopause as it helps to maintain the metabolism and keep the thyroid functioning at its optimum. Iodine is also present in the seaweed flakes, which supply other trace minerals too.

Both the peppers and tomatoes deliver a good degree of antioxidants, which carry huge anti-ageing and anti-cancer benefits.

SERVES 6–8
PREPARATION: about 15 minutes
COOKING: about 35 minutes, plus a few minutes' standing

2 tablespoons olive oil

2 onions, chopped

2 garlic cloves, finely chopped

2 peppers, preferably of different colours, deseeded and cut into thick strips

1 small head of fennel, cored and chopped, reserving any fronds to garnish

400 g / 14 oz tinned chopped plum tomatoes

Pinch of saffron strands (optional)

Freshly ground sea salt and black pepper

350 g / 12 oz long-grain rice

About 850 ml / 1½ pints miso broth (see page 176) or fish or shellfish stock (see page 177)

Handful of mixed seaweed flakes

225 g / 8 oz peeled cooked prawns

200 g / 7 oz canned mussels, drained

85 g / 3 oz pitted black olives

Lemon wedges, to serve

Heat the olive oil in a large deep frying pan or paella pan. When good and hot, sauté the onion until translucent. Add the garlic, pepper strips and fennel, and sauté briefly until just beginning to soften.

Add the tomatoes and saffron, if using. Season to taste and bring to the boil. Add the rice, stirring in well. Pour in the stock, sprinkle in the seaweed flakes and bring back to the boil again. Lower the heat, cover and simmer gently for about 20 minutes, until the rice is tender.

Take off the heat, mix in the prawns, mussels and olives, and adjust the seasoning. You might also want to add a little more stock or boiling water to moisten the paella – it should be neither sticky like a risotto nor dry like a pilaf. Cover and leave to stand for a few minutes until the seafood is thoroughly warmed through.

Serve garnished with the reserved fennel fronds, and accompanied by lemon wedges.

VEGETABLE MASALA

P ★★★ E ★ A ★★★

As well as making a nice change for a weekday meal, this also makes an unusual accompaniment to roast, baked or grilled fish for Sunday lunch. The vegetables offer a good supply of antioxidants and the miso broth, potatoes, carrots and broccoli are rich in phytoestrogens.

SERVES 4–6 as a main course
PREPARATION: about 25 minutes
COOKING: 30–40 minutes

225 g / 8 oz potatoes, cut into bite-sized cubes

Freshly ground sea salt and black pepper

2 teaspoons coriander seeds

1 teaspoon fennel seeds

1 teaspoon cumin seeds

3 tablespoons olive oil

2 large onions, chopped

3–4 garlic cloves, finely chopped

2–3 hot red chillies, deseeded and finely chopped

1-cm / ½-in piece of root ginger, finely chopped

225 g / 8 oz carrots, sliced at an angle

½ cauliflower, separated into bite-sized florets

175 g / 6 oz broccoli, separated into bite-sized florets and stalks cut into cubes

175 g / 6 oz green beans

400 g / 14 oz tinned chopped plum tomatoes

2 tablespoons tomato paste

1 tablespoon honey

300 ml / ½ pint miso broth (see page 176) or vegetable stock (see page 177)

2 teaspoons garam masala

2 tablespoons chopped coriander, plus more whole sprigs for garnish

First parboil the potatoes for about 10 minutes in plenty of boiling salted water. Drain and leave to cool. When they are cool enough to handle, cut them into bite-sized cubes.

Lightly crush all the spices and seeds using a mortar and pestle.

Heat 2 tablespoons of oil in a large heavy-based pan and, when hot, sauté the spices over a fairly high heat until they are aromatic and sizzling. Add the onions and sauté until they are just translucent. Add the garlic, chillies and ginger, and sauté for a minute or two more.

Add all the fresh vegetables and turn or shake over a moderate heat for a few minutes to coat them well in the oil and spices. Add the tomatoes with their liquid, the tomato paste, honey, broth or stock and season to taste. Stir well, cover and cook gently for about 15–20 minutes, until the vegetables are all just tender.

Heat the remaining oil in a small pan and cook the garam masala for 1–2 minutes. Stir into the vegetables, add the coriander and cook for 2–3 minutes. Serve garnished with coriander sprigs.

MASOOR DHAL WITH CABBAGE

P ★★★★★   E ★   A ★★★

Lentils, like chickpeas, supply all four isoflavones and so are an excellent source of plant hormones, together with the rice. The cabbage, as a cruciferous vegetable, gives good anti-cancer protection by helping oestrogen to be excreted in its harmless form. The ginger is helpful for circulation and the powerful antioxidant, lycopene, comes from the tomatoes.

Serve this with basmati rice or Cinnamon Rice (see page 132), or with chapati or naan bread. (See photograph, page 23.)

SERVES 4
PREPARATION: about 30 minutes
COOKING: about 1¼ hours

225 g/8 oz masoor dhal (red split lentils), well rinsed
Good pinch of ground turmeric
3 tablespoons olive oil
1 teaspoon cumin seeds
3 garlic cloves, finely chopped
1 large onion, thinly sliced
1 hot red chilli, deseeded and finely chopped (optional), plus more sliced chillies for garnish
225 g/8 oz firm cabbage, finely shredded
Freshly ground sea salt and black pepper
½ teaspoon finely grated root ginger
400 g/14 oz tinned chopped plum tomatoes
½ teaspoon garam masala
1 tablespoon finely chopped coriander leaves, plus more whole leaves to garnish

Put the lentils in a large heavy pan, add 850 ml/1½ pints of fresh water and bring to the boil. Skim off any scum and stir in the turmeric. Turn down the heat, partially cover and leave to simmer gently, stirring from time to time.

While the lentils are cooking, heat the oil in a large frying pan over a moderate heat. Add the cumin seeds and sauté for a few seconds. Add the garlic and toss until just beginning to colour, then add the onion, chilli and cabbage. Stir-fry for a few minutes until the cabbage begins to colour and become crisp. Season and set aside.

When the lentils have been cooking for 1¼ hours, stir in the ginger, tomatoes and garam masala, with seasoning to taste. Cook over a moderate heat, partially covered, for a further 10 minutes or so.

Add the contents of the pan together with the coriander to the lentils, heat gently and serve, garnished with whole coriander and sliced chilli.

STORECUPBOARD MIXED BEAN AND TOMATO CASSEROLE

P ★ ★ ★ ★ ★   E ★ ★   A ★ ★ ★

Another warming and nourishing dish, this casserole gives plenty of phytoestrogens from the different mix of beans and the miso broth. The seaweed flakes provide vital trace minerals and the tomatoes the antioxidant lycopene, which is thought to ward off cardiovascular problems and degenerative eye conditions. Try the casserole with a crisp green salad.

SERVES 4
PREPARATION: about 15 minutes
COOKING: about 1 hour

2 tablespoons olive oil
2 large onions, chopped
2–3 garlic cloves, finely chopped
1–2 small hot red chillies, deseeded and finely chopped (optional)
100 ml/3½ fl oz red wine (optional)
Two 400 g/14 oz tins of chopped plum tomatoes
5 tablespoons tomato paste
300 ml/½ pint miso broth (see page 176) or vegetable stock (see page 177)
Large handful of mixed dried seaweed flakes
2 teaspoons dried thyme
2 teaspoons dried oregano
1 teaspoon dried sage
2 tablespoons flat-leaved parsley, chopped
Freshly ground sea salt and black pepper
400 g/14 oz tinned butter beans, drained
400 g/14 oz tinned or bottled cannellini beans, drained
400 g/14 oz tinned red kidney beans, drained

FOR THE TOPPING:
25 g/1 oz wholemeal breadcrumbs
25 g/1 oz peanuts, crushed
15 g/½ oz butter, melted

Preheat the oven to 180°C/350°F/Gas 4.

Heat the oil in a large flameproof casserole and, when hot, sauté the onions until just translucent. Add the garlic and chillies (if using) and sauté for a minute or two more. Add the wine (if using) and boil to reduce to a sticky residue. Then add the tomatoes with their liquid, the tomato paste, broth or stock, seaweed flakes and the dried and fresh herbs. Season to taste, mix well and simmer for about 15 minutes.

Spread a quarter of this mixture in the bottom of an ovenproof casserole, then layer up the beans, with a layer of tomato mixture between them. Finish with a layer of tomato mixture.

Mix together the topping ingredients and sprinkle evenly over the casserole. Bake until the topping is nicely browned, about 30 minutes.

VEGETABLE, BEANSPROUT AND TOFU STIR-FRY

P ★ ★ ★ ★ ★   E ★   A ★ ★ ★

Stir-fries are so easy to make and so very good for you, as the nutrients from the vegetables are not lost through heavy cooking. A varied mix of phytoestrogens is provided in this tasty stir-fry, with the tofu, broccoli, mushroom and beansprouts. There is also a plentiful supply of anti-ageing and anti-cancer antioxidants in the peppers, mange-tout, sweetcorn, broccoli and tomatoes. (See photograph opposite.)

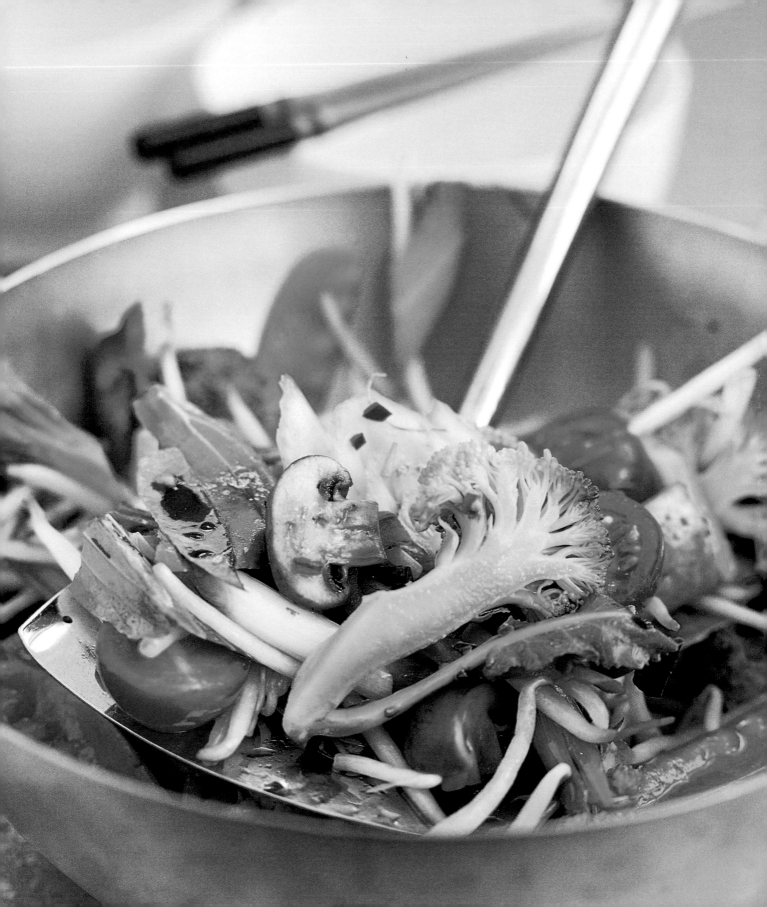

SERVES 4

PREPARATION: about 15 minutes

COOKING: 10–15 minutes

About 2 tablespoons olive oil

*6 spring onions, cut across at an angle into
2.5-cm/1-in lengths*

1–2 red chillies, deseeded and finely chopped

285g/10oz tofu, cut into small bite-sized cubes

*2 sweet peppers (preferably red and yellow), deseeded
and cut into strips*

100g/3½oz mange-tout peas

100g/3½oz baby sweetcorn, halved

100g/3½oz broccoli, separated into bite-sized pieces

100g/3½oz cherry tomatoes

100g/3«oz chestnut mushrooms, halved

*100g/3½oz bok choy, choy sum or other Chinese leaves,
torn into large pieces*

200g/7oz beansprouts

Soy sauce to taste

Small splash of sesame oil

Heat the oil in a large wok until quite hot and then
add the spring onion and chillies. Stir-fry until
wilted and aromatic, about 2–3 minutes. Remove
with a slotted spoon and keep warm in a bowl.

Add the tofu and stir-fry until well coloured.
Again remove from the wok with a slotted spoon
and keep warm in the bowl.

Add the peppers, peas, sweetcorn and broccoli
and stir-fry for 2 or 3 minutes, then add the
tomatoes and mushrooms and stir-fry for 2 more
minutes. Remove and keep warm in the bowl.

Add the Chinese leaves to the wok and stir-fry
until wilted. Now return all the other items from
the bowl to the wok, together with the beansprouts.
Turn over a moderate heat for a minute or so,
seasoning to taste with the soy sauce and sesame oil,
until all is well warmed through. Serve at once.

TOFU AND MUSHROOM STROGANOFF

P ★★★★ E ★ A ★

Stroganoff is a lovely way to vary the taste of
tofu by marinating it so it can pick up all the
different flavours.

The rice or noodles will supply additional
phytoestrogens to those in the tofu and the
mushrooms, and the onions are believed to help
prevent bones from thinning.

SERVES 4–6

PREPARATION: about 10 minutes,
plus 30 minutes' marinating

COOKING: 15–20 minutes,
plus cooking rice or noodles

1 tablespoon dark soy sauce

1 tablespoon no-added-sugar Worcestershire sauce

2 tablespoons sweet paprika

Freshly ground sea salt and black pepper

225g/8oz soft tofu, cut into bite-sized strips

3 tablespoons olive oil

2 large onions, halved and sliced

15g/½oz butter

225g/8oz chestnut mushrooms, sliced

300ml/½ pint sour cream or crème fraîche

Lemon juice to taste

*Boiled basmati rice or fresh egg noodles,
to serve*

Well ahead of time, mix the soy and Worcestershire
sauces with half the paprika and some seasoning in a
shallow bowl.

Toss the tofu strips in the mixture and leave to
marinate for at least 30 minutes, stirring from time
to time.

Heat 2 tablespoons of the oil in a large frying pan and sauté the onions with the paprika until the onions are translucent.

Add the marinated tofu with any liquid left in the bowl and continue to sauté until the tofu is well browned all over and the onions lightly browned. Transfer the contents of the pan to a bowl and keep warm.

Heat the remaining oil in the pan with the butter and sauté the chestnut mushrooms until well coloured. Add the contents of the bowl back to the pan, together with the sour cream or crème fraîche. Mix well, season to taste with salt, pepper and lemon juice, and bring back to a simmer for a minute or two.

Serve with rice or noodles.

HOPPIN' JOHN WITH GREENS

P ★★★★   E ★   A ★★★

This is a version of a homely Mississippi bean dish that is said to bring good fortune if eaten on New Year's Day. Served with a mixed salad, it makes good eating any day of the year.

The black-eyed beans, known as peas in the States, are high in phytoestrogens. To pack even more nutrients into this dish, cook the beans with a strip of kombu (seaweed), as mentioned in the introduction to the recipes (see page 44).

The dark green leafy vegetables offer excellent quantities of antioxidants as well as other vitamins and minerals such as iron.

SERVES 4–6

PREPARATION: about 20 minutes, plus overnight soaking

COOKING: 1¼–1½ hours, plus 1 hour's standing

285 g/10 oz black-eyed beans

1 large onion, chopped

2 garlic cloves, finely chopped

Pinch of dried red pepper flakes

1 bay leaf

2 large handfuls of mixed seaweed flakes

Freshly ground sea salt and black pepper

225 g/8 oz collard greens, spring greens or kale, shredded

225 g/8 oz long-grain brown rice

25 g/1 oz butter

Cayenne pepper

Soak the black-eyed beans overnight in cold water to cover generously.

Next day, drain and rinse them, then measure them by volume in a measuring jug. Put them in a large pan with 3½ times their volume of fresh cold water. Bring to the boil and boil hard for 5 minutes, then leave to stand for 1 hour.

Add the onion, garlic, red pepper flakes, bay leaf, half the seaweed flakes and black pepper to taste. Bring to the boil again, lower the heat, cover and simmer for another 1–1½ hours, until the beans are tender.

Towards the end of the cooking time, cook the greens in a separate pan of salted water with the remaining seaweed flakes until just tender, drain well and keep warm.

At the same time, cook the long-grain rice in a separate pan of salted water until just tender but still *al dente*. Drain well and then fluff over a very low heat.

When the black-eyed beans are cooked, mash some of them a little with a fork, then stir in the greens, rice and butter. This gives a mixed consistency. Adjust the seasoning to taste with pepper, salt and cayenne, and heat through gently before serving.

BOSTON BAKED BEANS

P ★★★★   E ★   A ★

It's important to give yourself a variety of legumes to supply your phytoestrogen needs. This time they are contained in the haricot or navy beans. The seaweed flakes provide iodine, vital for healthy thyroid function and its anti-cancer benefits. Antioxidants are found in the tomato ketchup and red wine.

SERVES 6 (with second helpings all round)
PREPARATION: about 10 minutes, plus overnight soaking
COOKING: 3–4¾ hours, plus making the ketchup

450 g/1 lb dried haricot beans, preferably navy beans, rinsed and soaked overnight

25 g/1 oz butter

2 tablespoons olive oil

3 large onions, chopped

4 garlic cloves, finely chopped

25 g/1 oz mixed dried seaweed flakes

600 ml/1 pint tomato ketchup (see page 178)

4 tablespoons maple syrup

4 tablespoons dark molasses

3 tablespoons no-added-sugar Worcestershire sauce

3 tablespoons red wine

1 tablespoon cider vinegar

2 teaspoons mustard powder

Freshly ground sea salt and black pepper

Chopped parsley, to garnish (optional)

Bread or toast, preferably wholemeal, to serve

Drain the beans, rinse well again and put in a large heavy pan. Cover generously with fresh (unsalted) water and bring to the boil. Reduce the heat and simmer gently until just tender, 50–90 minutes, depending on the beans. When cooked, drain the beans, reserving the cooking water.

Preheat the oven to 150°C/300°F/Gas 2.

Heat the butter and oil in a large flameproof casserole over a moderate heat and sauté the onions and garlic in it until translucent.

Stir the seaweed, tomato ketchup, syrup, molasses, Worcestershire sauce, wine, cider vinegar and mustard into 175 ml/6 fl oz of the reserved bean cooking liquid. Then stir this into the casserole, bring to a simmer and mix in the beans thoroughly. Season to taste.

Cover and cook in the oven for 2–3 hours, scraping up the bottom layer from time to time to prevent burning and adding a little water if at any time it seems too dry. Uncover the casserole for the last 30 minutes or so to brown the top and ensure that the beans are thick and syrupy.

Serve immediately, served on toast or accompanied by good bread and garnished with some chopped parsley, if you like.

PIZZA MARINARA

P ★★★   E ★★★★   A ★★

This is definitely not your average pizza, as it contains phytoestrogens in the form of soya flour and fennel. (See photograph opposite.) The oily fish give the Omega 3 essential fatty oils which are so important for healthy skin and hair as well as keeping the hormones in balance.

Eating raw onions has been found to reduce cholesterol by increasing the 'good' (HDL) cholesterol. Both raw and cooked onions can help to prevent blood clots, and so defend against heart attacks and strokes. The seaweed rounds off the nutritious ingredients with its store of vital trace minerals.

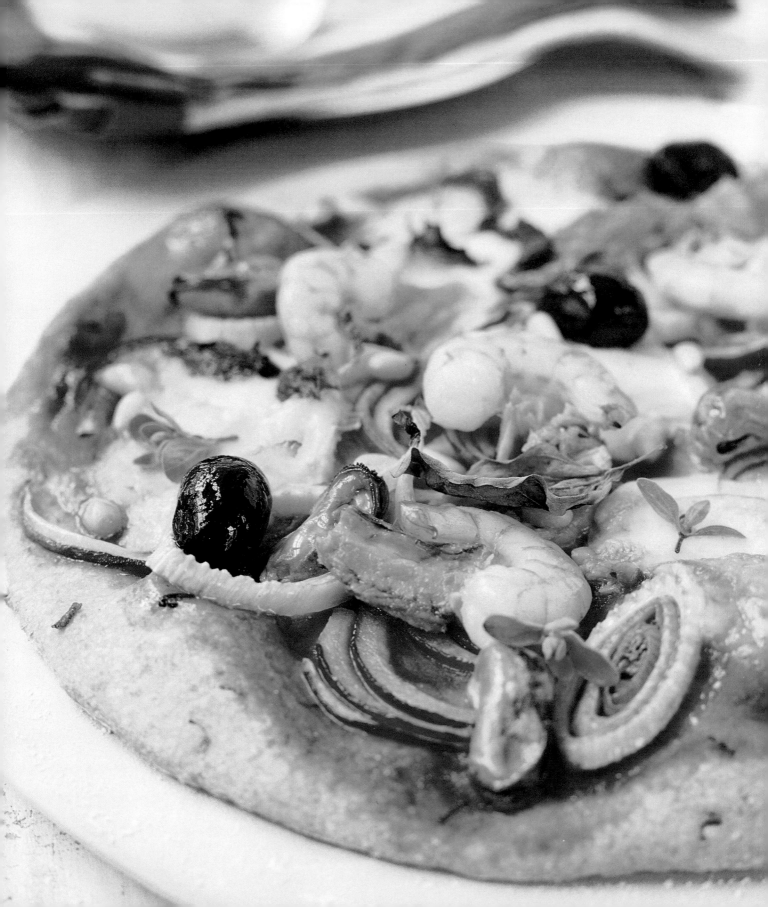

As this pizza dough, containing wholewheat and soya flours, is inevitably a little heavier and more 'bready' than ordinary pizza dough, to get a nice crisp result it helps to use a specially made pizza tin with holes all over it to allow hot air to get to the dough. Try also to get the centre of the pizza base to be thinner than the edges.

SERVES 4–6 (makes one 30-cm/12-in diameter round pizza)

PREPARATION: about 45 minutes, plus 2½ hours' rising

COOKING: 18–20 minutes, plus 5 minutes' resting

FOR THE DOUGH:

265 ml/9½ fl oz water, warmed to blood heat

1 teaspoon honey

20 g/¾ oz fresh yeast, or 1 sachet of easy-blend dried yeast

250 g/9 oz Italian type 00 or strong white flour, plus more for dusting

125 g/4½ oz wholewheat flour

125 g/4½ oz soya flour

4 tablespoons extra-virgin olive oil

A few turns of freshly ground sea salt

Good handful of mixed seaweed flakes

FOR THE TOPPING:

350 g/12 oz passata or tinned plum tomatoes, puréed

Freshly ground sea salt and black pepper

Soy sauce

Balsamic vinegar

1 small bulb of fennel, cored and cut into bite-sized pieces

1 small red onion, halved and sliced

1 fresh (preferably buffalo) Mozzarella cheese, about 100 g/3½ oz, cut into slices

Half 100 g/3½ oz tin of mussels, drained

85 g/3 oz frozen cooked and peeled large prawns

Half 100 g/3½ oz tin of tuna in oil, drained and separated into small bite-sized pieces

Juice of ½ lemon

A few sprigs of basil

Handful of pitted black olives

5 quails' eggs (optional)

55 g/2 oz pine nuts

To make the yeast, put 3 tablespoons of the water and the honey in a large bowl and stir in the fresh yeast (if using easy-blend yeast, add it to the flour, never to wet ingredients). Mix the dough to a cream. Add 4 tablespoons of the Italian or strong white flour and mix to a soft dough (add a little more flour or water, if necessary). Knead for 3 minutes, sprinkle with more flour, then cover with a tea towel and leave to rise for 30 minutes.

Once risen, gently rewarm the remaining water to blood heat. Sift the remaining flours into the bowl, pour over a little water and pinch the dough, flour and water together to mix.

Gradually add more water, pinching together, until all the water is added, then repeat with 1 tablespoon of oil. When you have a softish ball of dough, make a dent in the top and add some salt, the seaweed flakes and another tablespoon of oil.

Now knead everything together until it is no longer sticky and the inside surface of the bowl is clean. Toss the dough and stretch it into a flat shape on a floured work surface. Drizzle on one more spoonful of oil and knead, then repeat, kneading for a good minute more. The dough is ready when it feels silky, but not too silky. Put the dough back in the bowl and cut a big cross in the top with a knife. Sprinkle with flour, cover with a tea towel and leave in a warm place to double in size, about 2 hours.

Preheat the oven to 250°C/475°F/Gas 9 or to its highest setting. Lightly flour the work surface again and knead or roll the risen dough on it for a few minutes, then roll it out to a round just big enough to line a 30-cm/12-in diameter round pizza tin (if you haven't got one, just make the pastry round on a large baking sheet). Press it evenly into the tin, so it is slightly thinner in the middle and leaving it heavily indented with your fingertips. Trim the edges, if necessary, and prick it all over with a fork.

Prepare the topping: season the tomato passata or purée with salt and pepper, and a dash each of soy sauce and balsamic vinegar. Spread it all over the pizza base, taking it quite close to the edge. Scatter the fennel and onion over that, then arrange the cheese slices here and there. Dot the mussels, prawns and tuna about. Sprinkle the seafood with lemon juice and the cheese with a dash of balsamic vinegar. Put some sprigs of basil on top of each cheese slice and scatter the olives here and there. If you are using them, break the eggs into little recesses among the other ingredients. Finally, season the topping well and scatter with the pine nuts.

Bake immediately for 18–20 minutes, until puffed and golden. Don't open the oven for the first 15 minutes or you'll let the heat out and your base won't be as crisp. Let it rest out of the oven for about 5 minutes before serving it, cut into wedges.

PASTA WITH ROAST GARLIC AND PINE NUTS

P ★★   E ★★★   A ★

The garlic and parsley as well as the wholemeal pasta in this dish give plenty of plant hormones. The linseed oil and the pine nuts supply good amounts of both Omega 3 and 6 essential oils.

You don't have to roast garlic especially for this dish; next time you are roasting anything, simply pop a few extra heads in the oven. Use some of them then, as they will go well with anything you are cooking (provided it is savoury, of course), and keep three in the fridge for this dish. You really don't need Parmesan with this dish, but you can serve it if you wish; do, however, offer a fresh green or tomato salad.

SERVES 4
PREPARATION: about 20 minutes
COOKING: about 40 minutes

3 large heads of garlic
About 2 tablespoons olive oil
450g/1lb (preferably wholemeal) pasta, such as tagliatelle, tagliarini or linguine
Freshly ground sea salt and black pepper
1 tablespoon linseed oil
65g/2oz pine nuts, lightly toasted
3 tablespoons chopped flat-leaved parsley or basil, plus more whole sprigs to garnish

Preheat the oven to 180°C/350°F/Gas 4. Leaving the heads of garlic intact, remove the papery outer skin. Brush the heads all over with olive oil and arrange in a small ovenproof dish that is just big enough to hold them in a single layer. Add a splash of water and cover with an ovenproof lid. Bake for about 30 minutes, until tender. Allow to cool until they can be handled.

Towards the end of the roasting time, start cooking the pasta in a large pan of boiling salted water, until the pasta is *al dente*, ie soft but still offering some resistance when you bite into it.

While the pasta is cooking, take one of the garlic heads and squeeze the softened garlic from all its cloves. Purée this with the linseed oil and remaining olive oil. Carefully peel the rest of the garlic cloves to keep them intact. Mix these with the garlic purée, pine nuts, parsley or basil and seasoning.

When the pasta is ready, drain well, tip it into the sauce and toss to dress uniformly. Garnish with some parsley or basil sprigs and serve immediately.

HERBY TOFU AND OAT BANGERS WITH NUTTY MASH

P ★ ★ ★ ★ ★   E ★ ★   A ★

There is such a variety of goodness in this one delicious dish. Plant hormones are available from the tofu, hummus (made from chickpeas), parsley and potatoes. The oatmeal is another source of phytoestrogens and is especially good for maintaining healthy cholesterol levels as well as supplying excellent levels of fibre, which helps to prevent unwanted 'old' oestrogens circulating in the body.

You can make a nice 'gravy' for these bangers by thickening some miso broth (see page 176) with arrowroot and serving the bangers with some fried onions, into which some sesame seeds and/or linseeds have been mixed.

MAKES 8–10

PREPARATION: about 30 minutes, plus 10 minutes' chilling

COOKING: 20–25 minutes

200g/7oz oatmeal, plus more for coating

250g/9oz silken tofu

Handful of fresh thyme

Large bunch of fresh chives

Large handful of flat-leaved parsley

Large handful of mixed dried seaweed flakes

3 tablespoons hummus (see page 59 or preservative-free ready-made)

150g/5oz mature Cheddar cheese, coarsely grated

1 tablespoon honey

2 tablespoons soy sauce

1 tablespoon no-added-sugar Worcestershire sauce

1 egg

Freshly ground sea salt and black pepper

Flour, for dusting

Olive oil, for frying

FOR THE NUTTY MASH:

1kg/2¼lb potatoes

2 tablespoons walnut oil

2 tablespoons olive oil

Freshly ground sea salt and black pepper

85g/3oz almonds, finely chopped

3 tablespoons flat-leaved parsley, chopped

Put all the ingredients for the bangers in a food processor with generous seasoning to taste and process until cohering together. Do not over-mix or the bangers will be too dense.

With floured hands, form the mixture into small tennis ball-sized spheres, roll on a coating of more oats and then pat these out into sausage shapes (try to give them four long flat sides as this will make the frying easier). Chill for about 10 minutes. (If you had trouble getting good shapes, they will be easier to shape after chilling.)

While they are chilling, cook the potatoes for the mash in boiling salted water until tender. Drain well and steam dry in the hot pan. Keep warm.

Fry the bangers gently in hot olive oil, turning regularly, until well browned on all sides, about 15–20 minutes in all.

Mash the dried potatoes, adding the walnut and olive oils and seasoning. Finish by mixing in the chopped nuts and parsley.

Serve at once, accompanied by the nutty mashed potatoes.

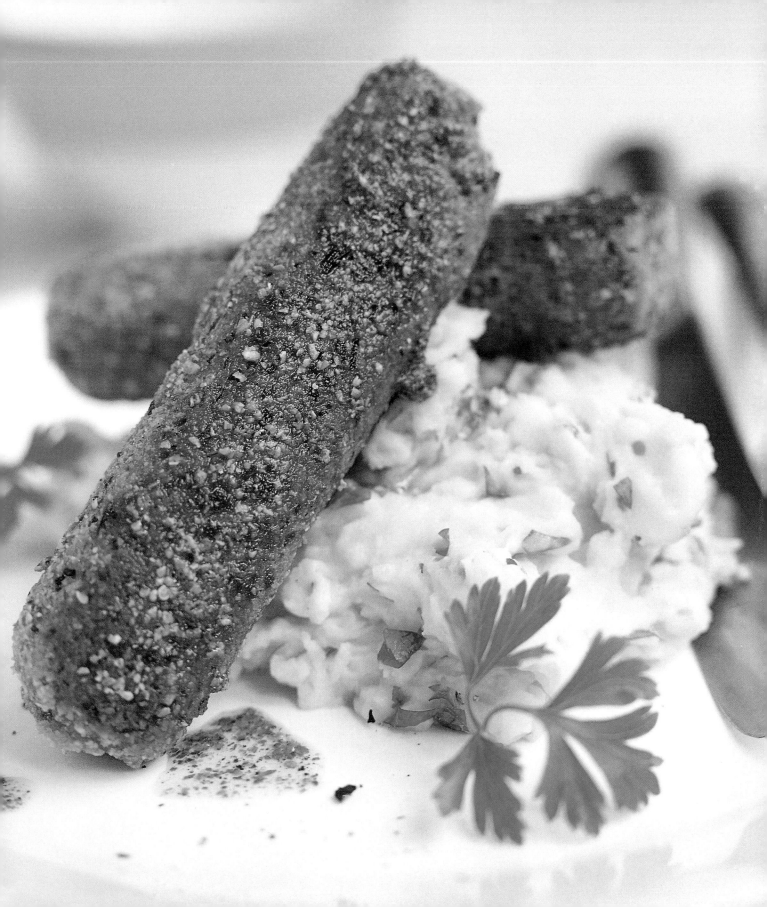

MIXED VEGETABLE STEW WITH HERB DUMPLINGS

P ★★★★   E ★★   A ★★★★

Stew is always a real comfort on cold days, and so rich in flavour. This warming dish has plenty of powerful antioxidants: beta-carotene in the carrots and lycopene in the tomatoes. Phytoestrogens are supplied by the miso broth, seeds, soya milk and soya flour. If chilli tends to bring on hot flushes in you, omit it.

SERVES 6–8
PREPARATION: about 35 minutes
COOKING: about 1¼ hours

2 tablespoons olive oil

450g/1lb onions, chopped

3–4 garlic cloves, finely chopped

2–3 small hot red chillies, deseeded and finely chopped (optional)

225g/8oz carrots, thickly sliced at an angle

225g/8oz potatoes, cut into bite-sized cubes

225g/8oz leeks, thickly sliced at an angle

100ml/3½ fl oz red wine (optional)

400g/14oz tinned chopped plum tomatoes

300ml/½ pint miso broth (see page 176) or vegetable stock (see page 177)

1 bouquet garni

1 tablespoon fennel seeds

1 tablespoon celery seeds

2 tablespoons sesame seeds

Freshly ground sea salt and black pepper

175g/6oz shelled or frozen peas

175g/6oz green beans

225g/8oz courgettes, thickly sliced at an angle

FOR THE HERB DUMPLINGS:

40g/1½ oz cold butter, shredded in a grater

100g/3½ oz self-raising flour, plus more for dusting

1 tablespoon soya flour

Freshly ground sea salt and black pepper

About 6 tablespoons finely chopped mixed fresh herbs such as parsley, chives, thyme and basil

About 5 tablespoons soya milk

Heat the oil in a large flameproof casserole and, when hot, sauté the onions until just translucent. Add the garlic and chillies and sauté for a minute or two more. Add the carrots, potatoes and leeks and toss to coat. Add the wine (if using) and boil to reduce it to a sticky residue.

Next add the tomatoes with their liquid, the broth or stock, bouquet garni and the seeds. Season well and bring to the boil. Reduce the heat, cover and simmer gently (or cook in the oven at 150°C/300°F/Gas 2) for about 45 minutes.

Towards the end of that time, prepare the dumplings: in a mixing bowl, rub the butter roughly into the sieved flours with seasoning to taste until the mixture resembles coarse crumbs. Stir in the herbs and add just enough of the milk to mix to a soft dough. Using floured hands, form the dough into about 18–20 small balls.

After the 45 minutes, take the casserole out of the oven (if it is in there) or remove from the heat. Remove and discard the bouquet garni. Favouring the potatoes above all, carefully transfer about one-quarter of the contents of the casserole to a food processor and purée until fairly smooth, but not too smooth.

Pour the puréed mixture back into the casserole and stir in the remaining vegetables, then float the dumplings on top. Bring back to a simmer on the stove, cover again and then either continue to simmer or return to the oven for a further 20 minutes.

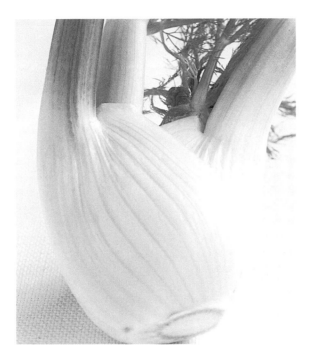

Side dishes

BRAISED FENNEL

P ★★★★   E ★   A ★★

This wonderfully tasty, phyto-packed dish makes the most exquisite accompaniment to baked or roast fish. All those phytoestrogens come from the fennel, miso broth, carrot and garlic, and the carrot provides some of the important antioxidant, beta-carotene.

SERVES 4
PREPARATION: about 15 minutes
COOKING: about 2 hours

2 large heads of fennel
Freshly ground sea salt and black pepper
2 tablespoons olive oil
1 small onion, sliced
1 carrot, finely diced
1–2 garlic cloves, finely chopped
Juice of ½ lemon
300 ml/½ pint miso broth (see page 176) or vegetable stock (see page 177)
1 bouquet garni
1 tablespoon coriander seeds, crushed
Handful of mixed dried seaweed flakes
15 g/½ oz butter

Trim the fennel, reserving any fronds. Cut the heads lengthwise in half and cut out the woody cores. Parboil the pieces of fennel for about 10 minutes in boiling salted water. Drain well and set aside.

Heat the oil in a heavy flameproof casserole or pan big enough to take the fennel in a single layer. Sauté the onion and carrot in it for a minute or two, until softened. Then add the garlic and sauté for a minute more.

Stir in the lemon juice, stock, bouquet garni, coriander seeds and seaweed and add seasoning to taste. Cover and bring slowly to the boil. Lower the heat and simmer, still covered, for about 10 minutes.

Arrange the fennel pieces, cut side down, on the bed of vegetables. Dot with the butter, cover again tightly and cook very, very gently for about 1–1½ hours, until the fennel is quite tender.

Remove the bouquet garni and serve garnished with the reserved fennel fronds.

Variation: you can also braise the fennel in an oven preheated to 180°C/350°F/Gas 4. An interesting variation on this dish is to mix the fennel with young celery hearts.

COLCANNON

P ★★   E ★   A ★★★★

This version of the classic of the Irish kitchen is beautifully tasty as well as being full of goodness.

The soya milk and potatoes are the phytoestrogen providers in the recipe. If you use cabbage, you will be giving yourself extra cancer protection since the vegetable helps unwanted oestrogen to be excreted in its harmless form. This is especially important at the menopause. Otherwise, green vegetables supply excellent levels of antioxidants.

It is traditional in Ireland not to mix in the melted butter, but to pour it into a recess made in the middle of the mixture: you then dunk forkfuls of the mash in the butter as you eat it. Using spring onions as the green element gives you the other traditional mashed potato dish, champ.

SERVES 6

PREPARATION: about 15 minutes

COOKING: about 20 minutes

1kg/2¼lb floury potatoes, peeled and chopped

1kg/2¼lb cabbage, kale or other leafy green vegetable, shredded

300ml/½ pint soya milk

50g/2oz butter, plus more for frying

Freshly ground sea salt and black pepper

Cook the potatoes and greens in separate pans of boiling salted water until quite soft, about 20 minutes. Drain well.

Mash the potatoes until smooth, then beat in the greens and the milk, followed by the butter and seasoning to taste.

Variation: you can also form the mixture into small cakes and fry these in butter until crisp and brown on both sides. For an extra phyto boost, add to the mash a spoonful or two of sesame seeds, linseeds or poppy seeds.

BRUSSELS SPROUTS
WITH PEANUT SAUCE

P ★   E ★ ★   A ★ ★ ★

For those for whom years of soggy overcooked sprouts have produced a complete lack of respect for this Cinderella of veg, try this way with them and rediscover their natural crunch and flavour.

Brussels sprouts, like cabbage and cauliflower, belong to the cruciferous family of vegetables which helps protect against oestrogen-dependent cancers of the breast and womb. This is because the indoles contained in the sprouts help to metabolise oestrogen and eliminate it safely from the body. Brussels sprouts also have good amounts of antioxidants, in the form of vitamin C and beta-carotene. Lastly, the pine nuts are full of essential oils.

This dish makes a good accompaniment for the Tofu and Mushroom Stroganoff (see page 106), the Herby Tofu and Oat Bangers (see page 112), or the Storecupboard Mixed Bean and Tomato Casserole (see page 104).

SERVES 4

PREPARATION: about 10 minutes

COOKING: 7–8 minutes, plus making the sauce

500g/1lb 2oz Brussels sprouts

Freshly ground sea salt

2 tablespoons soy sauce

1 recipe quantity peanut sauce (see page 182)

2 tablespoons olive oil

4 tablespoons pine nuts, lightly toasted

Cook the Brussels sprouts in boiling salted water for about 5–6 minutes, until just tender. Drain well.

Mix the soy sauce into the peanut sauce and set aside.

Heat the oil in a wok or large frying pan, then quickly stir-fry the sprouts for 2 minutes. Remove from the heat and stir half the peanut sauce into the pan.

Transfer to a warmed serving dish, spoon over the remaining sauce and sprinkle with the pine nuts.

ROAST ROOT VEG WITH HERBS, SEEDS AND GARLIC

P ★ ★   E ★   A ★ ★ ★ ★

Serve these luxurious vegetables alongside whole fish for Sunday lunch – or even Christmas – and you have a banquet.

The vegetable feast also gives you plenty of the free radical busters, antioxidants. Carrots in particular contain excellent amounts of the powerful antioxidant, beta-carotene, which is effective in delaying ageing and preventing cancer. Unusually, a cooked beetroot contains more nutrients than a raw one. These include good levels of vitamin C and potassium, which helps to control water retention.

Phytoestrogens are supplied by the carrots and potatoes, and walnuts are especially good for the heart because of their effect on cholesterol.

SERVES 4

PREPARATION: about 20 minutes

COOKING: about 1 hour

1.5kg/3¼lb mixed root vegetables, including as many of the following as possible: potatoes, parsnips, carrots, celeriac, baby turnips, beetroots and shallots

1 head of garlic

100ml/3½fl oz olive oil

1 tablespoon honey

2 tablespoons sesame seeds

Several sprigs each of thyme and rosemary

Freshly ground sea salt and black pepper

55g/2oz walnut halves

Preheat the oven to 200°C/400°F/Gas 6 and bring a large pan of salted water to the boil. Prepare the root vegetables, leaving any that are 'baby', or bite-sized, whole. Cut the potatoes into largish chunks and the carrots into smallish pieces (as they take longer to cook), making the rest a fairly uniform size in between. Separate the garlic into cloves, but leave them unpeeled.

Parboil all the vegetables except the garlic in the boiling water for about 5 minutes only. Drain well and return to the hot pan to steam dry.

In a small bowl, mix the oil with the honey, sesame seeds, herbs and lots of seasoning. Add this to the pan of vegetables with the garlic and walnuts and toss to coat them all well in the mixture.

Turn the contents of the pan out into a roasting pan and roast for 45–60 minutes, shaking or stirring from time to time to help them cook uniformly, until all the vegetables are tender. (If they seem to be browning too fast before getting tender, cover them with a lid for the last part of cooking.)

BRAISED RED CABBAGE WITH WINTER FRUIT

P ★   E ★   A ★ ★ ★ ★

Red cabbage is a superb ingredient as it is valuable in the fight against cancer as well as possessing antioxidant benefits. Phytoestrogens are present in the cinnamon, caraway seeds and apples. The seaweed flakes will give you valuable nutrients, including iodine for a healthy thyroid. There are also plenty of different bioflavonoids contained in the array of fruits included here. (See photograph opposite.)

If chestnuts are added to the dish, they will increase the antioxidant levels since chestnuts contain good amounts of vitamin E. Try the dish with the Herring with Oatmeal (see page 90), or the Roast Nut-coated Cod (see page 144).

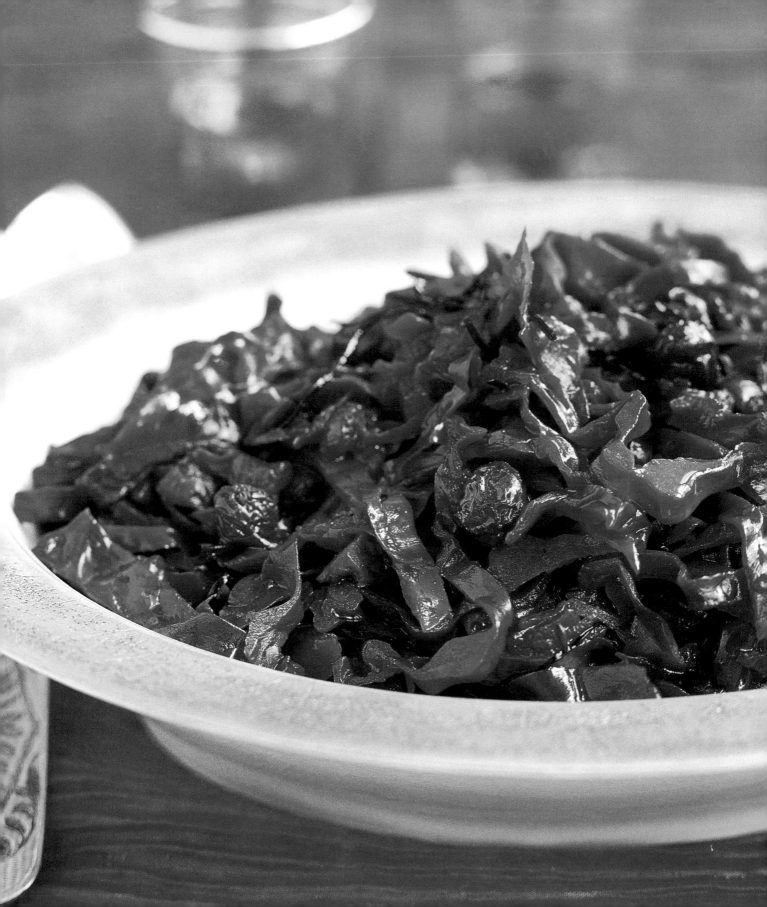

SERVES 4–6

PREPARATION: about 15 minutes

COOKING: about 1¼ hours

15 g/½ oz butter

1 tablespoon olive oil

1 large onion, finely chopped

½ head of red cabbage (about 675 g/1½ lb), shredded

5 tablespoons cider vinegar

5 tablespoons dry red wine (optional)

Large pinch of ground cinnamon

Handful of mixed seaweed flakes

1½ tablespoons honey

Juice and grated zest of 1 small orange

Juice and grated zest of 1 small lemon

1 large tart apple, diced

115 g/4 oz seedless raisins

85 g/3 oz cranberries

1 teaspoon caraway seeds

Freshly ground sea salt and black pepper

Melt the butter with the oil in a large heavy-based pan or casserole, add the onion and cook gently until translucent.

Add the remaining ingredients with plenty of seasoning and mix well. Bring to a simmer, cover tightly and cook over a gentle heat for about 1¼ hours, stirring from time to time. (You may also have to add a little more water if it shows any signs of getting too dry at any time.)

Adjust the seasoning if necessary before serving.

Variation: add some chopped boiled chestnuts to make this into a meal in itself.

COURGETTE AND SAFFRON SPAGHETTI

P ★   E ★★   A ★★★

Just a small portion of courgettes (100 g/3½ oz) provides you with more than a quarter of your daily needs of vitamin C. The pine nuts give you good amounts of essential oils. You have to make this dish (see photograph opposite) at the very last minute to preserve its freshness and texture.

SERVES 4

PREPARATION: about 5 minutes

COOKING: about 5 minutes

25 g/1 oz butter

1 tablespoon olive oil

Pinch of saffron strands

Freshly ground sea salt and black pepper

600 g/1 lb 5 oz (5–6) medium to large (but not too big) young firm courgettes, unpeeled, but topped and tailed

55 g/2 oz pine nuts, lightly toasted

Melt the butter with the oil in a large heavy frying pan over a gentle heat. Once melted, stir in the saffron and plenty of salt and pepper (enough to provide seasoning for all the courgettes once they are added). Leave over the gentlest of heats while you prepare the courgettes.

Using the shredding disc of a food processor, shred the courgettes into long spaghetti-like strands.

Turn up the heat under the frying pan and, when the butter is hot, tip in all the courgette strands. Working quickly, toss them with a pair of spatulas or spoons, so that all the strands are coated in the saffron butter and warmed through (you don't want them to cook all that much or they will overcook).

Serve immediately, topped with the pine nuts.

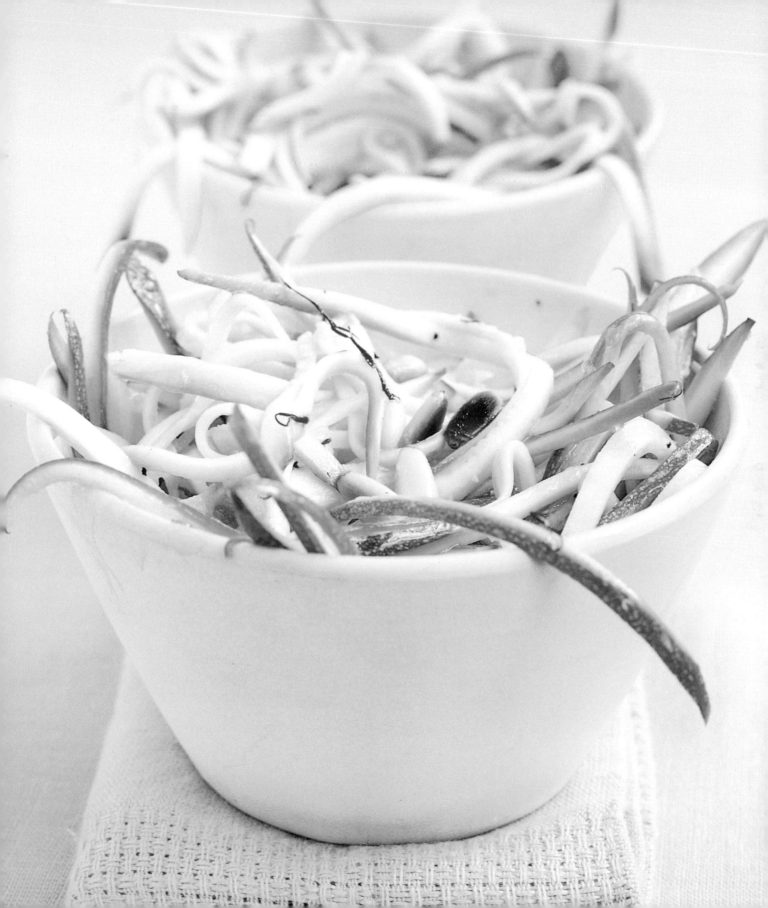

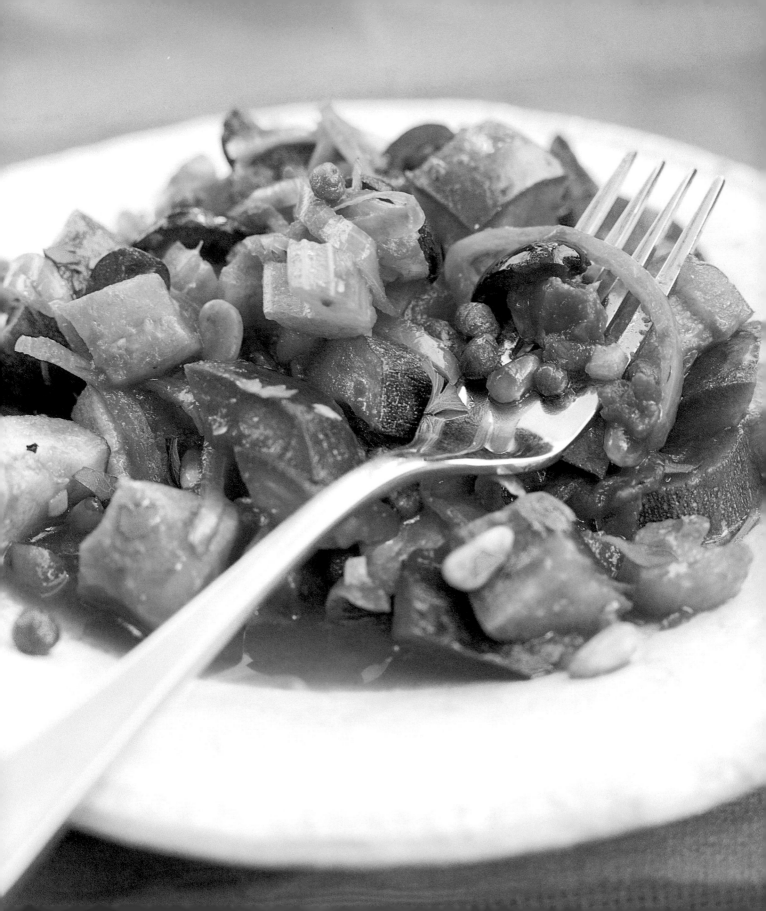

CAPONATA

P ★★★★   E ★★★★   A ★★★★

Caponata (see photograph opposite) is the Sicilian version of ratatouille. In its home country it is a classic accompaniment to fried or grilled fish, squid or prawns. Served cold, it makes an excellent starter.

The dish comprises such a wide mix of ingredients that nearly everything in this recipe will benefit your health in one way or another. Good levels of antioxidants to prevent cell damage and premature ageing are derived from the tomatoes and courgettes. Essential oils are provided by the pine nuts and anchovies. The fennel gives you good amounts of plant hormones, with extra help from the parsley and garlic. And lastly, the cider vinegar and honey mix is very beneficial because it helps you absorb more calcium from this dish.

SERVES 4
PREPARATION: about 20 minutes, plus 20 minutes' draining
COOKING: about 2 hours, plus cooling (if serving cold)

2 aubergines, cut into 1-cm/½-in cubes
Freshly ground sea salt and black pepper
About 3 tablespoons olive oil, plus more for greasing
1 large onion, sliced
2 large garlic cloves, finely chopped
225g/8oz tinned chopped plum tomatoes, liquid drained but reserved
1 bouquet garni
2 tablespoons tomato paste
1 tablespoon honey
3 tablespoons cider vinegar
2 large courgettes, halved lengthwise and then sliced
16 anchovies, rinsed, drained and cut into strips
55g/2oz pine nuts, lightly toasted
55g/2oz salted capers, rinsed and drained
2–3 celery stalks, thinly sliced
85g/3oz pitted black olives, cut into strips
About 2 tablespoons finely chopped flat-leaved parsley

Sprinkle the aubergine generously with salt and leave to drain in a colander for about 20 minutes. Rinse well and pat dry.

Preheat the oven to 180°C/350°F/Gas 4 and grease a large ovenproof casserole with some of the oil.

Heat the remaining oil in a large pan and sauté the onion until translucent. Add the garlic and cook for a minute or two more.

Stir in the tomatoes, bouquet garni and tomato paste. Bring to a simmer and cook gently for about 20 minutes, until the mixture is reduced to a thick paste. Discard the bouquet garni, stir in the honey and vinegar and simmer for a minute more.

Stir in the aubergines, courgettes, anchovies, pine nuts, capers, celery and olives. Season to taste.

Transfer to the prepared casserole, cover and bake for about 1½ hours, or until all the vegetables are quite tender. Stir from time to time to prevent sticking; if the contents of the casserole at any time look too dry, try adding some of the reserved tomato liquid.

Serve warm or cool, sprinkled with finely chopped parsley.

VEGETABLE TABBOULEH

P ★ ★ ★ ★ ★   E ★ ★ ★ ★   A ★ ★ ★ ★

This version of the classic Lebanese salad contains seven different sources of phytoestrogens in the one dish – linseeds, bulgur wheat, garlic, carrots, courgettes, broccoli and peas – which shows how easy it is to include them in your diet. The linseed oil provides a good helping of essential fatty acids, which are crucial for lubricating joints and keeping your skin and hair healthy. The tomatoes are full of the antioxidant lycopene, which is protective against cancer and heart disease.

The tabbouleh (see photograph opposite) is an excellent accompaniment to grilled fish and vegetables. It also makes a fine first course (serve it with Cos lettuce heart leaves as scoops). It is particularly good for barbecues and picnics as it keeps its taste and texture without the worry of it going soggy, as dressed leaf salads do.

SERVES 6–8

PREPARATION: 20 minutes, plus 40 minutes' soaking

COOKING: about 1 minute

175 g/6 oz bulgar wheat

1 tablespoon olive oil

1 tablespoon linseed oil

Juice of 3 lemons

2 garlic cloves, very finely chopped

Freshly ground sea salt and black pepper

2 large carrots

2 courgettes

Small head of broccoli

115 g/4 oz shelled peas

Small bunch of mint, finely chopped, reserving a few whole leaves to garnish

Large bunch of flat-leaved parsley, finely chopped reserving a few leaves to garnish

225 g/8 oz ripe juicy tomatoes, skinned (see page 50), stalks removed and diced

½ cucumber, diced

1 tablespoon golden linseeds

4–5 spring onions, chopped

Put the bulgar in a large bowl and cover well with warm water. Leave for about 20 minutes to swell and soften. Drain thoroughly, squeezing to remove excess moisture, and place in a large serving bowl.

Mix the oils with the juice of 2 of the lemons and the garlic. Season this dressing to taste and pour it over the bulgar. Mix well and leave for about 20 minutes more.

Put a large pan of salted water on to boil. Dice the carrots, courgettes and broccoli to about the same size, just a little larger than the largest of the peas. Put the peas and the diced vegetables in a blanching basket and, when the water is boiling rapidly, lower into the water for 1 minute only. Refresh in a bowl of cold water and then drain well.

When ready to serve, mix the chopped mint and parsley into the salad, together with most of the tomatoes, the cucumber, the linseeds, the drained blanched vegetables and about two-thirds of the spring onions. Adjust the seasoning with more salt, pepper and lemon juice, if necessary (it should taste quite sharp).

Garnish with the remaining tomatoes and spring onions and the reserved whole mint leaves and parsley leaves.

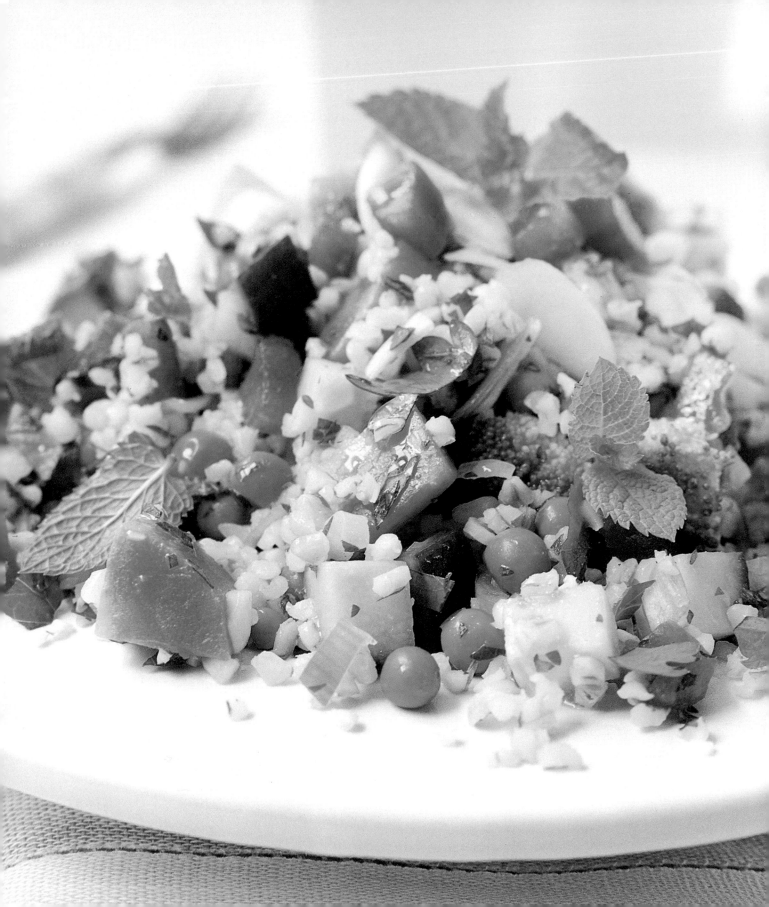

CAESAR SALAD

P ★　　E ★ ★ ★ ★　　A ★

This version of the American classic is a perfect summer salad that goes well with many robustly flavoured dishes as well as making a great first course. It has a wonderful mix of essential fatty acids from the linseed oil, anchovies and walnuts. Eggs are packed full of essential vitamins and minerals and the garlic is beneficial, both as a source of phytoestrogens and also as a booster to the immune system.

SERVES 4

PREPARATION: about 20 minutes, plus overnight infusing

COOKING: 1½ minutes (for the egg), plus making the croûtons

1 egg

1 large head of Cos lettuce

Freshly ground sea salt and black pepper

115g/4oz Parmesan cheese

55g/2oz walnut halves, lightly toasted and chopped

Garlic croûtons (see page 52)

FOR THE DRESSING:

4 tablespoons olive oil

2 tablespoons linseed oil

2 large garlic cloves, thinly sliced

Large pinch of mustard powder

6 anchovy fillets, rinsed, drained and finely chopped

½ teaspoon no-added-sugar Worcestershire sauce

3 tablespoons cider vinegar

Juice of 1 small lemon

The day before, put the oils for the dressing in a small bowl with the garlic slices and leave at room temperature to infuse with the garlic flavour.

Next day, when ready to serve, boil the egg for 1½ minutes only. Cool under cold running water. Shred the lettuce into a salad bowl, season well and scoop the contents of the egg shell over the leaves.

Grate half the Parmesan. In a bowl, mix all the dressing ingredients including the garlic oil (discard the slices of garlic or use them elsewhere) and the grated Parmesan. Sprinkle the dressing over the leaves and toss well. Add in the walnuts and croûtons and toss again.

Finish by shaving the remaining Parmesan into strips over the top of the salad.

PARSLEY SALAD

P ★ ★ ★　　E ★ ★ ★ ★　　A ★ ★ ★

It is important that you eat a variety of phytoestrogens and that you do not come to rely on just one source, such as soya. Parsley is yet another way to feed yourself these important substances. The dressing is also excellent for your health as it contains both linseed and olive oil as well as antioxidants from the tomatoes and carrot.

This refreshingly green-tasting salad (see photograph opposite) makes an ideal accompaniment to roast and grilled fish. It can also be served as a first course, topped with shavings of best-quality Parmesan cheese. For a more substantial dish you could try adding anchovies, or even crumbled goats' cheese.

This salad is based on a famous dish made by Australian chef Gay Bilson, whose original version is very concentrated and contains chopped anchovies. She serves little spoonfuls of it on her own cayenne biscuits to go with a welcoming glass of champagne.

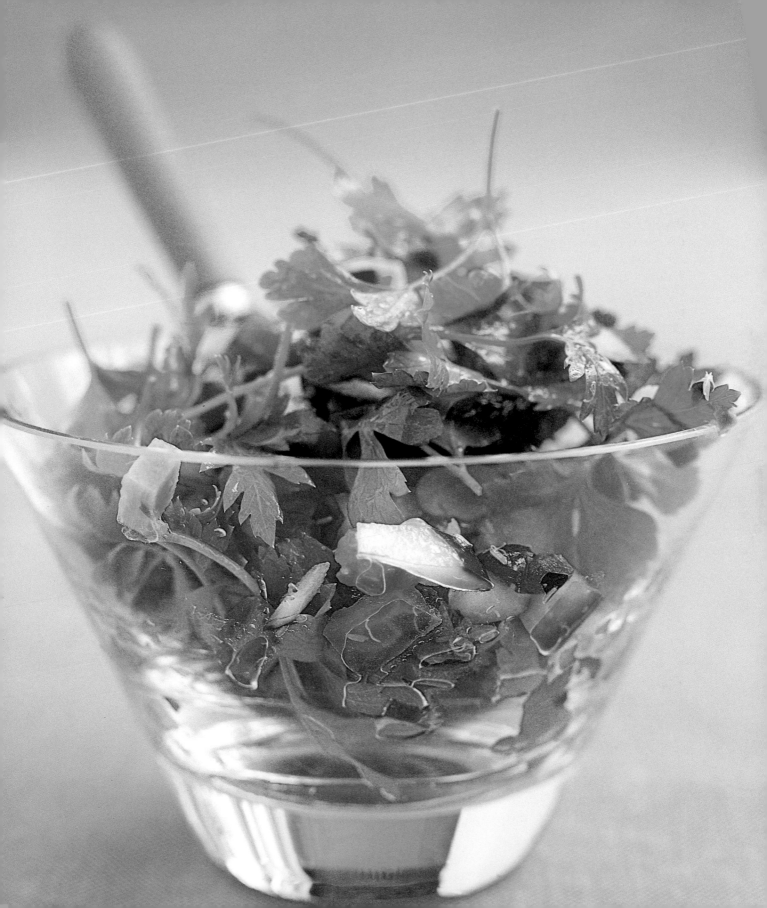

SERVES 4

PREPARATION: about 25 minutes

About 200g/7oz flat-leaved parsley, leaves separated and all stalks removed

FOR THE DRESSING:

115g/4oz pitted black olives, finely chopped

1 large red onion, finely chopped

2 garlic cloves, finely chopped

About 1 tablespoon salted capers, rinsed and finely chopped

4 ripe plum tomatoes, skinned (see page 50), deseeded and diced small

1 large carrot, diced small

About 125 ml/4½fl oz extra-virgin olive oil

2 tablespoons linseed oil

Juice and grated zest of 2 lemons

Freshly ground sea salt and black pepper

Mix all the ingredients for the dressing in the bottom of a glass salad bowl, with seasoning to taste.

Just before serving, throw the parsley leaves into the bowl and toss to coat them well.

FATTOUSH

P ★★★★   E ★★★   A ★★★

Fattoush is a wonderful Syrian bread salad (see photograph opposite). Once again linseeds (and their oil) prove their worth. Not only do they contain phytoestrogens – as do the parsley, garlic and soya yoghurt – but also essential fatty acids. These essential oils help to keep your hormones in balance and your skin and hair soft. Both the peppers and tomatoes are rich in antioxidants and so help disarm free radicals.

SERVES 4

PREPARATION: about 25 minutes

COOKING: about 5 minutes (for toasting the bread)

2 large flat pitta breads

Juice of 2–3 large lemons

1 large red onion, finely chopped

6 large ripe vine-ripened tomatoes, chopped

1 cucumber, diced

2 small peppers, preferably of different colours, deseeded and finely diced

1 garlic clove, finely chopped

100 ml/3½fl oz olive oil

2 tablespoons linseed oil

About 6 tablespoons finely chopped flat-leaved parsley

About 2 tablespoons finely chopped coriander leaves

About 2 tablespoons finely chopped mint leaves

1 tablespoon golden linseeds

Freshly ground sea salt and black pepper

Pomegranate seeds, to garnish (optional)

Soya yoghurt, to serve (optional)

Open out the pitta breads and toast them lightly on both sides, then break them up into bite-sized pieces.

Just before you want to serve the salad, put all the ingredients, including the pitta, in a large glass salad bowl and toss well. Season to taste and add more lemon juice if necessary.

Serve immediately, garnished with pomegranate seeds if you choose and with soya yoghurt on the side.

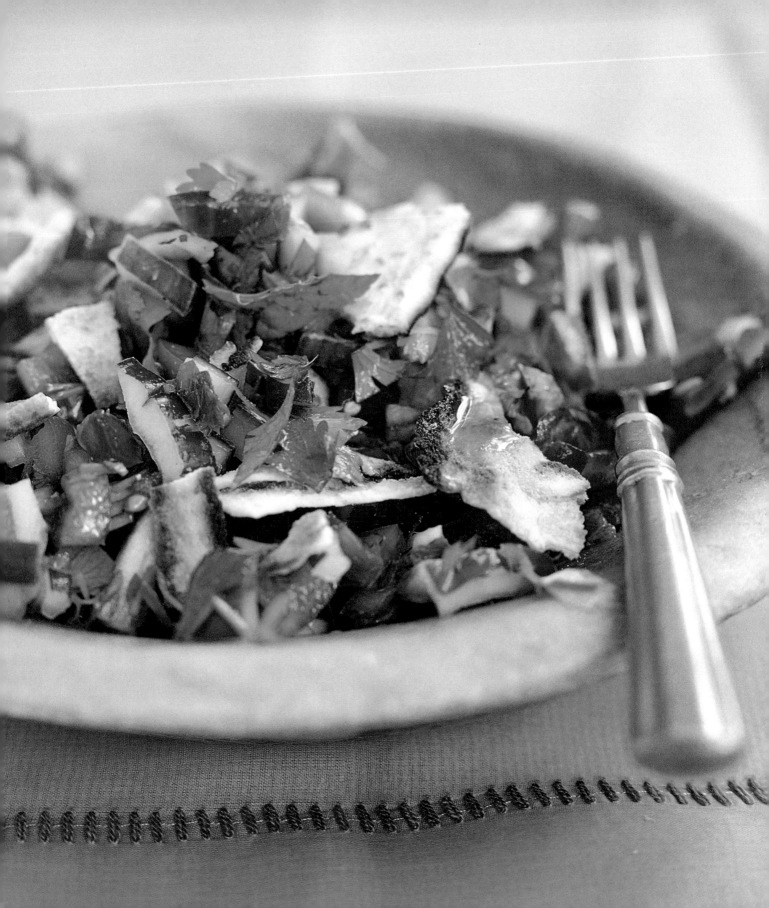

CARROT AND CELERIAC REMOULADE

P ★★   E ★★   A ★★

This refreshing and tangy salad is delicious with cold fish and seafood. It also makes a good first course for a summer's meal.

Celeriac, which is part of the celery family, has good amounts of potassium – an excellent mineral for helping with water retention. The carrots contain the antioxidant beta-carotene as well as plant hormones. The linseeds likewise are an important source of phytoestrogens, as well as carrying essential oils.

SERVES 6–8

PREPARATION: about 20 minutes, plus making the mayonnaise

COOKING: 2 minutes

1 small celeriac

3–4 carrots

FOR THE REMOULADE DRESSING:

1 recipe quantity mayonnaise (see page 179)

1 tablespoon grainy mustard, or more to taste

1 tablespoon golden linseeds

2 gherkins, very finely diced

2 tablespoons chopped herbs, including flat-leaved parsley, chives, chervil and tarragon, plus more for garnish

2 tablespoons capers, chopped

Freshly ground sea salt and black pepper

Dash of Tabasco

Juice of 1–2 lemons, according to taste

Bring a large pan of salted water to the boil. Grate the vegetables into long strands and put these into the boiling water. Boil for 2 minutes only, then drain and plunge immediately into a bowl of cold water to stop the cooking process. Drain thoroughly and pat dry using a clean cloth or paper towels.

While the vegetables are cooking and draining, make the rémoulade sauce by mixing all the ingredients together and seasoning to taste with salt, pepper, Tabasco and lemon juice.

In a large bowl, mix the vegetables into the sauce, adjusting the seasoning if necessary, and sprinkle with more herbs to serve.

AUSTRIAN BEAN SALAD WITH TOFU DRESSING

P ★★★★★   E ★★★   A ★

The delicious tofu dressing and unusual marriage of apples and gherkins with the beans makes for an extremely tasty and pretty dish (see photograph opposite).

The various beans give you plentiful supplies of fibre as well as phytoestrogens, with extra amounts coming from the apples and potatoes. The dressing is made with beneficial linseed oil as well as olive oil, which is good for a healthy heart.

The bean salad goes very well with the Deluxe Kebabs (see page 136) but is also very satisfying as a starter on its own. If you are cooking the beans yourself, it is important to remember not to salt the pot until about halfway through cooking or the skins will toughen. Make sure you dress the drained beans while they are still warm so that the dressing really soaks in. For advice on cooking beans, see the Introduction to the Recipes (page 44).

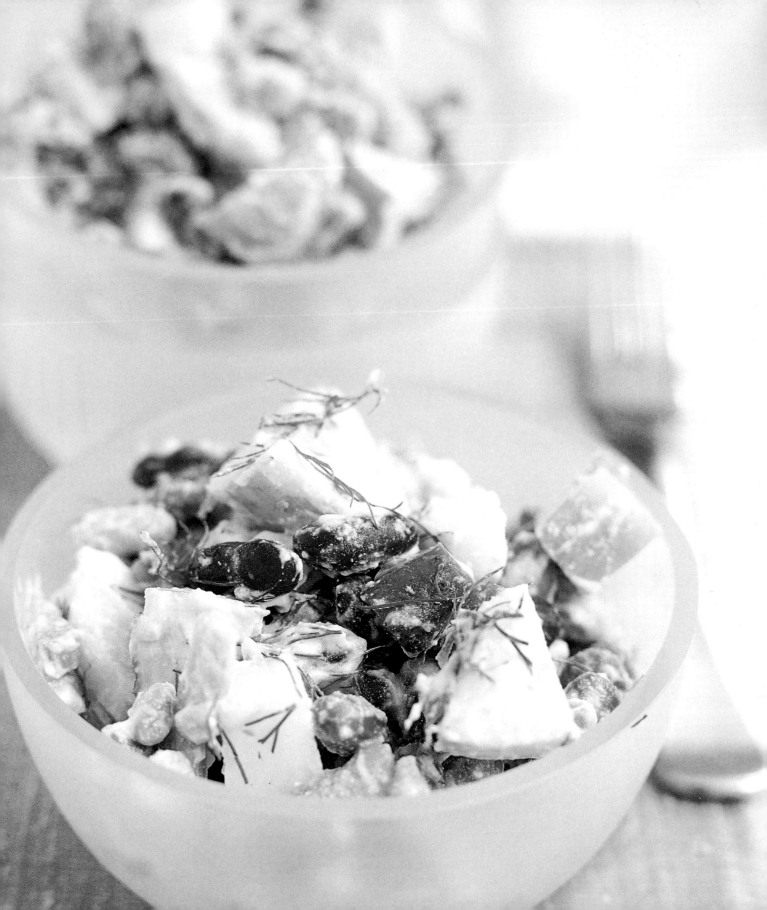

SERVES 4–6

PREPARATION: about 15 minutes,
plus cooking the potatoes and possibly the beans

175 g/6 oz tinned or cooked red kidney beans

175 g/6 oz tinned or cooked flageolet beans

175 g/6 oz tinned or cooked borlotti or cannellini beans

115 g/4 oz cooked waxy potatoes, diced

2 sharp firm eating apples, cored and diced

85 g/3 oz sweet gherkins, finely diced

*1 tablespoon dill or fennel fronds, chopped, plus more
for garnish*

FOR THE TOFU DRESSING:

250 g/9 oz tofu

3 tablespoons cider vinegar

2 tablespoons olive oil

1 tablespoon linseed oil

1 teaspoon English mustard

1 tablespoon honey

Freshly ground sea salt and black pepper

Make the tofu dressing by blending all the ingredients in a food processor until smooth and seasoning to taste.

Put all the other ingredients in a large, preferably glass, salad bowl and pour over the dressing. Toss lightly to mix so that all the ingredients are lightly coated in the dressing but are still identifiable.

Serve garnished with more dill or fennel leaves.

CINNAMON RICE WITH NUTS AND RAISINS

P ★★　　E ★★　　A ★

This is a lovely way to serve rice; for added benefits you can buy organic brown basmati rice. Rice is a source of phytoestrogens, as is the cinnamon. The almonds will provide you with some essential oils.

SERVES 6–8

PREPARATION: about 10 minutes,
plus 30 minutes' optional soaking

COOKING: about 10 minutes,
plus 10 minutes' standing

225 g/8 oz basmati rice

Freshly ground sea salt

7.5-cm/3-in piece of cinnamon stick

2–3 bay leaves

55 g/2 oz seedless raisins

2 tablespoons flaked almonds, lightly toasted

Rinse the rice thoroughly in a sieve and, if you have time, soak in plenty of fresh cold water for about 30 minutes.

Bring 450 ml/¾ pint of water to the boil in a large pan. Add salt to taste, the cinnamon stick and the bay leaves. Bring back to the boil and tip in the drained rice. Stir well, reduce the heat to the barest simmer, cover tightly and cook for 10 minutes.

Take off the heat and leave without touching the lid for another 10 minutes.

After 10 minutes, remove the cinnamon and bay leaves. Mix in the raisins and nuts and fluff up with a fork.

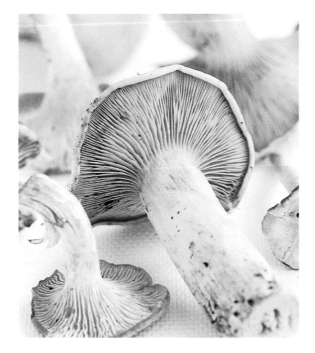

Weekend and special occasion dishes

GRILLED SEAFOOD SALAD

P ★★★★   E ★★★★   A ★★★★★

Not only will this colourful salad (see photograph opposite) transport you to the Mediterranean, but it will also give you a welcome nutritional boost. Plenty of selenium, a powerful antioxidant, is delivered by the shellfish in addition to other antioxidants from the green vegetables and tomatoes. There are excellent essential oils from the fish and linseed oil, plus phytoestrogens from the linseeds and fennel.

SERVES 6

PREPARATION: about 40 minutes, plus at least 1 hour's marinating

COOKING: about 25 minutes

225g/8oz prepared small squid

225g/8oz raw tiger prawns, shelled

225g/8oz medium scallops, halved across their thickness

225g/8oz small new potatoes

12 quails' eggs

1 large Cos lettuce or 3 Little Gems

1 head of radicchio

Small bunch of rocket

Small bunch of watercress

Several handfuls of various fresh herbs, such as flat-leaved parsley, chives, dill, chervil and coriander, plus more sprigs to garnish

1 cucumber

1 red onion, halved and sliced

1 small fennel bulb, cored and diced fairly small

225g/8oz cherry tomatoes, preferably Santa plum tomatoes, halved

55g/2oz salted capers, rinsed, drained and patted dry

115g/4oz pitted black olives, preferably garlic-flavoured

2 tablespoons golden linseeds (optional)

FOR THE MARINADE:

1 tablespoon fresh root ginger, finely chopped

1 garlic clove, finely chopped

2 tablespoons linseed oil

Juice of 2 limes

1 red chilli, deseeded and finely chopped (optional)

Freshly ground sea salt and black pepper

FOR THE DRESSING:

4 tablespoons extra-virgin olive oil

2 tablespoons walnut or linseed oil

1 tablespoon balsamic vinegar

1 tablespoon lemon juice

First prepare the seafood: if necessary, remove the squid heads (with tentacles) from the tubes and rinse all the seafood well (if they've been frozen, it's a good idea first to swish them about in large bowl of heavily salted water) and pat them dry. Remove the dark intestinal thread from the backs of the prawns and butterfly them open so that they lie flat.

Put all the ingredients for the marinade in a bowl, season to taste, add the seafood and toss well. Cover and chill in the refrigerator for at least 1 hour, stirring from time to time.

Cook the potatoes in boiling salted water until just tender. Drain and steam dry. Put another pan of water on to heat, add the eggs and bring to the boil. Allow to boil for 1 minute only and then rinse under cold water and drain.

Next prepare the fresh vegetables: shred the lettuce and radicchio leaves into the bottom of a large salad bowl together with the rocket and watercress leaves and all but a few sprigs of each of the herbs. Slice the cucumber lengthwise into 2 or 3 long slices and then cut these into long strips, finally cut across into 2-cm/¾-in chunks. Add the cucumber together with the onion, fennel and tomatoes to the bowl.

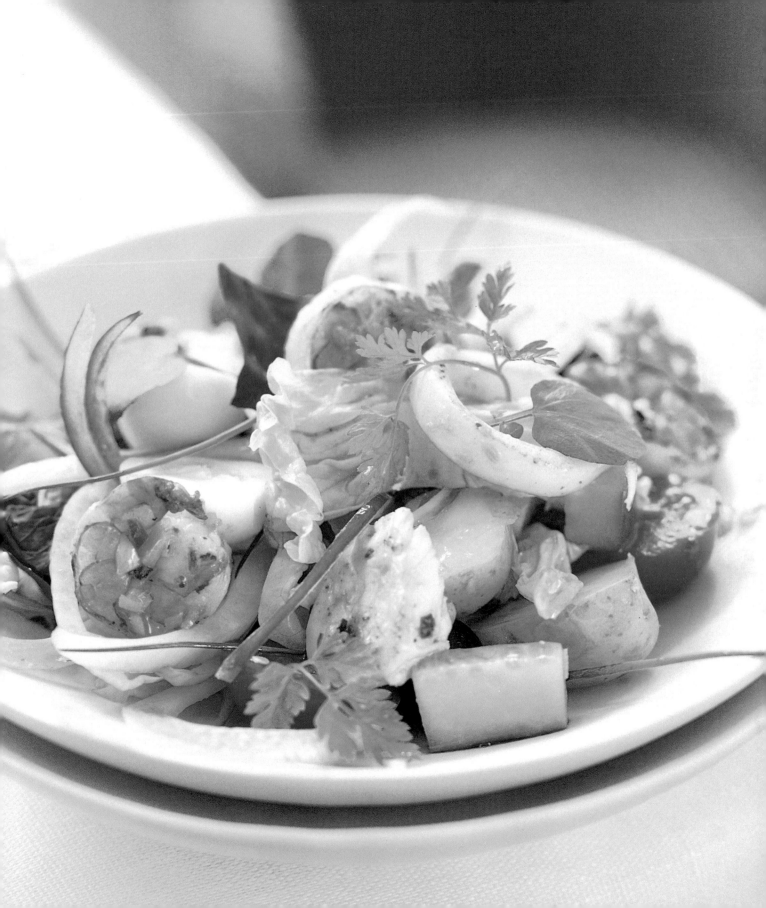

Preheat a hot ridged griddle pan. Make the dressing: blend all the ingredients and seasoning to taste. Shell the eggs and cut them in half.

Cut the potatoes into bite-sized chunks if necessary and add these to the salad with the capers, half the olives and the linseeds if using. Pour the dressing over the salad and toss well to mix. Taste and adjust the seasoning at this stage again.

Drain the seafood from the marinade and pat dry. Cook in batches on the hot griddle pan: starting with the squid, then the prawns and finishing with the scallops. The squid will need a minute or two on each side, as will the prawns, while the scallops literally need only about 15 seconds on each side. Try to get some nice sear marks from the hot pan ridges on the seafood but resist the temptation to overcook (which can happen in a matter of seconds with seafood and ruin it). As they are ready, scatter them over the tops of the salad.

Arrange the egg halves over the top of the salad, together with the remaining olives and herb sprigs.

DELUXE KEBABS

P ★★★★   E ★★   A ★★★★

These kebabs are a convenient and delicious way to serve tofu (an excellent source of phyto-estrogens), especially to people who may not have eaten it before. Prawns are a rich source of selenium and there are other antioxidants in the peppers and tomatoes. The sesame seeds also contain phytoestrogens and supply good quantities of essential fatty acids as well.

SERVES 6

PREPARATION: about 25 minutes, plus 3 hours' marinating

COOKING: about 15–20 minutes

6 red onions, quartered

200g/7oz firm tofu, cut into large bite-sized pieces

18 raw king prawns, shelled and deveined but with tails

6 large vine-ripened tomatoes, quartered

3 large peppers, preferably of different colours, quartered and deseeded

6 large Portobello mushrooms, cut into thick slices

12 bay leaves

Freshly ground sea salt and black pepper

25g/1oz sesame seeds

Lemon wedges, to serve

FOR THE MARINADE:

6 tablespoons olive oil

1 tablespoon soy sauce

2 tablespoons honey

3.5-cm/1½-in piece of root ginger, crushed

3 garlic cloves, crushed

2 tablespoons mirin (Japanese rice wine)

3 tablespoons oregano, chopped

1–2 red chillies, deseeded and finely chopped

Freshly ground sea salt and black pepper

Several hours ahead: mix all the marinade ingredients, except one-third of the oregano, in a large shallow bowl with seasoning to taste. Toss the red onions, tofu and prawns in the mixture. Cover and marinate in the refrigerator for at least 3 hours.

Preheat a hot grill or light a barbecue. Drain the onions, tofu and prawns from the marinade and thread them on 6 skewers interleaved with pieces of tomato, pepper, mushroom and bay leaves. Season if necessary and sprinkle with the sesame seeds.

Grill until well browned on all sides, occasionally basting with the marinade. Serve garnished with the remaining oregano and with lemon wedges.

Variation: For an Indonesian satay effect you could use peanut sauce as the marinade (see page 182).

GRILLED SCALLOPS WITH CHILLI JAM AND CREME FRAICHE ON A POTATO AND CARROT ROSTI

P ★   E ★★   A ★★

Shellfish like scallops are an excellent source of selenium, a powerful antioxidant. This dish (see photograph, page 6) has phytoestrogens via the carrots and potatoes. For centuries ginger has been used for its medicinal properties: it is good for the digestion and circulation, and can also help with inflammation – particularly useful at the menopause when one of the symptoms can be joint paints.

Scallops are fairly expensive items, so it is worth going the whole hog and paying that little bit extra for hand-dived scallops, which have a much better flavour and consistency. Ask your fishmonger or examine the shells if you can: hand-dived scallops will have good-looking intact shells, whereas the shells of dredged specimens will tend to look battered and chipped.

When cooking scallops in this way, remember to take them out of the fridge some time ahead of cooking; otherwise, with such brief cooking, you may find that although the outsides of the scallops are perfectly cooked the cold interiors remain cold.

SERVES 4
PREPARATION: about 30 minutes
COOKING: about 30 minutes, plus cooling

10–12 large fat scallops
A little olive oil, for brushing
125 ml/4½ fl oz well-chilled crème fraîche
Mixed leaves and herbs, to garnish (optional)

FOR THE CHILLI JAM:
Juice and pared zest of 1 lime
Juice and pared zest of 1 small orange
6 large thin slices of fresh root ginger
1–2 (according to taste) hot red chilli(es), halved lengthwise and deseeded
150 ml/¼ pint maple or date syrup

FOR THE ROSTI:
450 g/1 lb potatoes in their skins
450 g/1 lb carrots
Freshly ground sea salt and black pepper
1 tablespoon fennel seeds, crushed
1 tablespoon olive oil, plus more for greasing
25 g/1 oz butter

First make the chilli jam: cut all the zest, ginger slices and chilli halves into thin julienne strips. Put these in a small pan with the citrus juices and syrup, and stir over a low heat until simmering. Simmer for 3–4 minutes, stirring occasionally, and leave to cool.

Make the rösti: cook the potatoes and carrots in boiling salted water for 10 minutes, until almost soft. Remove from the pan and allow to cool. When cool enough to handle, peel away the potato skins and grate the flesh coarsely. Grate the carrots similarly. In a bowl, mix these together with some seasoning and the crushed fennel seeds.

Heat the oil and butter in a large frying pan until very hot. Put four oiled 10-cm/ 4-in pastry cutters in the pan and fill these with the mixture, packing it down well. Reduce the heat and cook gently for 10 minutes.

When the undersides are nicely crisped and browned, remove each rösti from the pan by slipping a spatula under it. Carefully ease it out of the cutter mould and return it to the pan with the cooked side uppermost. Continue to cook for a further 10 minutes until the other sides are browned in the same way.

While the rösti are cooking on their second side, preheat a very hot griddle pan. Cut the scallops into two thinner discs, brush them on both sides very lightly with oil and cook them on the very hot griddle pan over a high heat for about 30–45 seconds on each side – no more as they toughen quickly! – until nicely seared and just cooked through.

Put a rösti in the centre of each serving plate and spoon some crème fraîche in an uneven layer on top of each. Arrange the scallops on top of that and spoon the jam over them (you may have to warm it through again very slightly and/or let it down with a little more lime juice to get a 'jammy' consistency). Serve immediately, garnished with some leaves and herbs if you like.

JAMBALAYA

P ★★★   E ★   A ★★★★★

This is a version of the classic of Creole cuisine served in all Louisiana homes and restaurants (see photograph opposite). Plant hormones are offered by the miso broth, celery, rice, mushrooms, garlic and parsley. The prawns, peppers and tomatoes contain antioxidants and the seaweed flakes are rich in extra nutrients.

SERVES 4–6
PREPARATION: about 20 minutes
COOKING: about 1 hour

900 g/2 lb unpeeled prawns
850 ml/1½ pints partially made miso broth (see page 176), seafood or vegetable stock (see page 177)
2 tablespoons olive oil
1 onion, chopped
2 celery stalks, chopped
2 peppers, preferably of different colours, deseeded and chopped
3 garlic cloves, finely chopped
450 g/1 lb medium-grain rice
Two 450 g/14 oz tinned chopped plum tomatoes
450 g/1 lb chestnut mushrooms, sliced
2 red chillies, deseeded and chopped
2 teaspoons chopped fresh thyme (or 1 teaspoon dried), plus more whole sprigs to garnish (optional)
Handful of mixed seaweed flakes
Freshly ground sea salt and black pepper
Dash or two of no-added-sugar Worcestershire sauce
2 tablespoons chopped parsley, plus more whole leaves to garnish

Peel the prawns, removing the heads and tails. Drop all the trimmings into a pan with the broth (before adding the miso) or stock and simmer gently for 20 minutes to enhance the flavour. Strain the broth (having stirred in the miso) or stock and keep hot.

Heat the oil in a large heavy-based pan and sauté the onion, celery and peppers for a few minutes until softened. Add the garlic and sauté for a minute or two more.

Stir in the rice and turn until all the grains are shiny and well coated with the oil. Pour in all the stock and add the tomatoes with their liquid, the mushrooms and the chillies, thyme and seaweed. Bring to the boil, stir well and season to taste with salt, pepper and Worcestershire sauce. Cover tightly and leave to simmer very gently for 25 minutes.

Add the prawns and parsley, cover again and simmer gently for another 5 minutes, or until the prawns are nicely cooked through. Serve with more parsley leaves and more thyme sprigs if you like.

Variation: for a more elaborate garnish, keep some of the shrimp in the shell and poach them briefly in the broth or stock until just cooked, then reserve and dot around the top of the dish when serving.

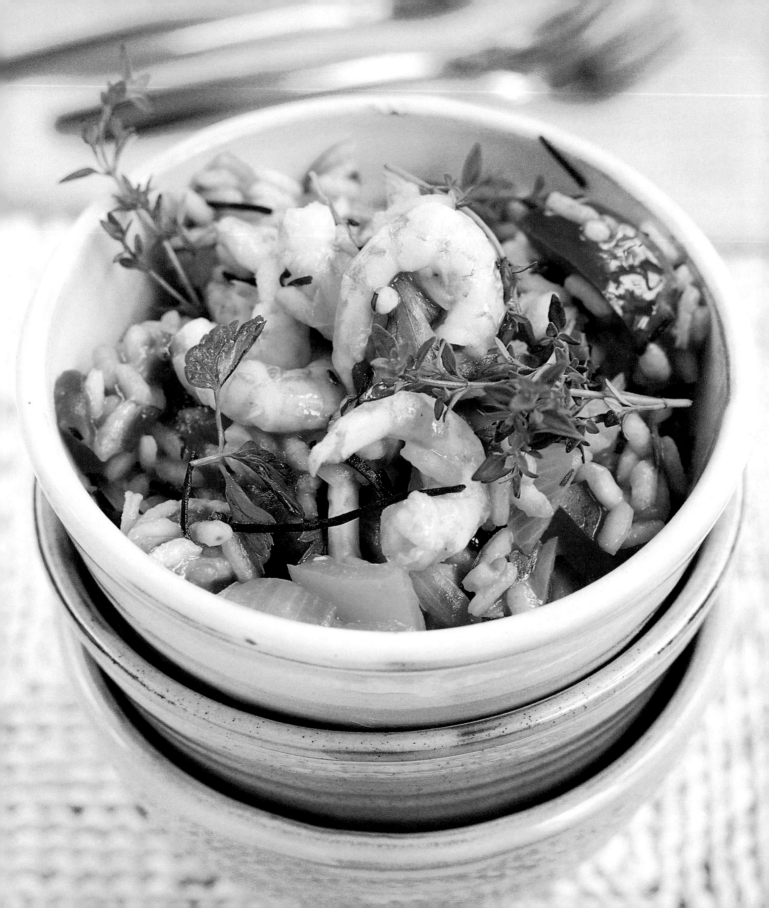

SUSHI ROLLS

P ★   E ★★★   A ★★

Seaweed suffers from a poor image: many
people think it is slimy and not very appealing.
Nori seaweed is quite different, in that it is very
thin and not at all slimy. Scientists have found
that seaweed is an excellent source of iodine,
which keeps the thyroid gland healthy, and that
seaweed can reduce cholesterol and help the
more efficient metabolism of fat. Eating sushi
(see photograph opposite) is an ideal
introduction to including seaweed in your diet,
and is also extremely healthy. Phytoestrogens are
available from the rice and essential oils from
the selection of fish and sesame seeds.

Nori, sushi rice, rice vinegar, mirin (Japanese
rice wine), pickled ginger and wasabi (a type of
Japanese horseradish) are sold in many health
food shops, in some better supermarket chains
and in specialist Japanese stores. Nori is usually
sold ready-toasted and perforated to make it
easier to cut through after rolling. If you can't
get hold of any nori, use a thick layer of lightly
toasted sesame seeds as the exterior coating –
the seeds will adhere to the rice. You will need a
bamboo sushi mat or a double layer of greaseproof paper on a tea towel to roll the sushi.

SERVES 6 (makes about 30)
PREPARATION: about 30 minutes
COOKING: about 20 minutes,
plus 10 minutes' standing

200g/7oz uncooked sushi rice
1 tablespoon salt
1 tablespoon mirin
3 tablespoons rice vinegar
1 tablespoon honey

55g/2oz sesame seeds, very lightly toasted in a dry pan
3 sheets of toasted nori (Japanese seaweed),
about 18×20cm/7×8in
3 tablespoons wasabi

FOR THE FILLINGS:
About 8–10 cooked shelled tiger prawns, butterflied open
About 115g/4oz mixed fresh crab meat
About 115g/4oz smoked salmon, cut into strips

TO SERVE:
Dark soy sauce
Pickled ginger
More wasabi

Put the rice in a sieve and rinse under running cold
water until the water runs clear, then drain well. Put
into a large pan, cover with 450ml/¾ pint cold
water and add the salt. Cover tightly, bring to the
boil and boil for 1 minute. Then turn the heat down
and cook gently for about 15 minutes, or until all
the water is absorbed and the rice is tender but still
has a slight resistance to the bite. Remove from the
heat and allow to stand, still covered, for 10 minutes.

Meanwhile, mix together the mirin, rice vinegar
and honey in a small pan and heat gently. Turn the
rice out into a large flat plate, sprinkle over the
sesame seeds and gently fold them and the dressing
into the rice with a wooden spoon. Cool the rice
by fanning it with a damp cloth. When the rice
stops steaming, cover it with the cloth.

Place a sheet of nori, with its shiny side down and
the perforations running vertically, on a sushi mat or
on a double layer of greaseproof paper set on a clean
tea towel. Spread one-third of the rice over about
two-thirds of the nori, leaving a clear margin at the
top, and smooth the surface.

Lay one filling in a horizontal line just off centre
towards the end closest to you, then smear a line of
wasabi across the remaining rice just up from the
filling. Pick up the mat or towel at the end closest to

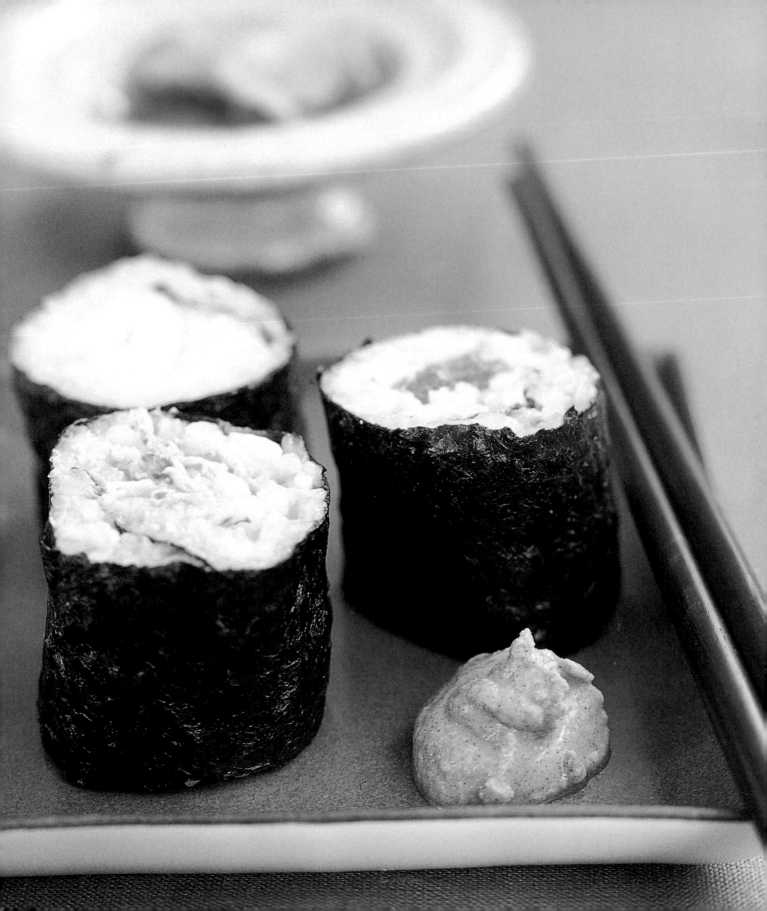

you, pull over the top, then push down gently with your fingers so that the end of the sushi roll tucks in and you can use the mat or towel to roll the whole thing up quite firmly, like a Swiss roll.

With a little water, dampen the bare edge of nori to help it stick. Tap the ends to neaten, leave to rest for a few minutes, then gently unroll the mat or greaseproof paper.

Slice the roll through the perforations or, if there aren't any, cut it into about 10 pieces. Repeat the process to make 2 more long rolls, each using a different filling, and cut each into pieces as before.

Serve accompanied by little bowls of soy sauce and side plates with some pickled ginger and a smear of wasabi for each person.

Variations: other suggestions for fillings include strips of cucumber, cooked spinach mixed with chopped anchovies, asparagus, avocado, salmon mousse, fresh tuna, or shiitake mushrooms lightly sautéed in olive oil.

WILD MUSHROOM RISOTTO

P ★★★   E ★   A ★★

The wonderfully versatile mushroom, which transforms so many dishes, has good levels of phytoestrogens. This is furthered by the plant hormones in the miso broth, rice and parsley in this dish. The shallots and garlic are from the *allium* family, which is known to boost the immune system and have anti-cancer qualities.

SERVES 4–6

PREPARATION: about 20 minutes, plus 20 minutes' soaking

COOKING: about 30 minutes, plus 5 minutes' standing

55 g/2 oz dried ceps

1.5 litres/2½ pints miso broth (see page 176) or vegetable stock (see page 177)

55 g/2 oz butter

4 tablespoons olive oil

6 shallots, finely chopped

3 garlic cloves, crushed

600 g/1 lb arborio rice

100 ml/3½ fl oz red wine (optional)

About 350 g/12 oz mixed fresh wild mushrooms (such as ceps, chanterelles, blewitts and trompettes de mort)

Freshly ground sea salt and black pepper

3 tablespoons parsley, chopped

85 g/3 oz Parmesan cheese, freshly grated

Rinse the ceps, put them in a small heatproof bowl and cover them with boiling water. Leave to rehydrate for about 20 minutes, drain, reserving the liquid, and chop quite finely.

Put the broth or stock in a pan and bring it to just below the boil. Keep it there throughout the operation.

Heat one-third of the butter and half the oil in a large heavy-based pan. Add the shallots and sauté until just translucent, then add the ceps and the garlic cloves and sauté for another 3–4 minutes.

Add the rice and stir around for a couple of minutes to coat well. Add the wine (if using) and boil it off (the pan gets really hot when you are stirring in the rice), then add the liquid from soaking the ceps and stir until it is absorbed.

Add a large ladleful of stock and stir until all the liquid is absorbed. Continue to add stock in the same way, for about 15–20 minutes, until the rice is tender but still firm to the bite and the risotto creamy and moist (if you run out of stock before the rice is tender, just add ladlefuls of boiling water).

Towards the end of this process, heat half the remaining butter and all the remaining oil in a large frying pan and cook each variety of mushroom separately, frying them until they just colour on each side. Transfer them to a warmed bowl as they are cooked. Season the cooked mushrooms really well and stir in the parsley.

When the risotto is ready, beat the remaining butter and the cheese into it. Stir in the mushrooms and adjust the seasoning if necessary. Cover and leave to stand for about 5 minutes before serving.

PAN-GRILLED DARNES OF SALMON ON PUY LENTILS

P ★★★★★   E ★★★★   A ★★

This is a wonderful succulent dish, packed with phytoestrogens from the lentils as well as excellent amounts of Omega 3 fatty acids from the salmon. The seaweed flakes give extra added value with their trace mineral content.

SERVES 4
PREPARATION: about 20 minutes, plus 1 hour's marinating and making the chive butter
COOKING: 35–45 minutes

4 darnes (thick boneless transverse cuts) of salmon, each about 175–225 g/6–8oz

2 tablespoons sesame seeds, lightly toasted

Chive Butter (see page 181), to serve

FOR THE MARINADE:

2 tablespoons olive oil

Juice of 1 lime

2 teaspoons soy sauce

1 teaspoon mixed peppercorns

1-cm/½-in piece of fresh root ginger, very finely chopped

FOR THE LENTILS:

1 tablespoon olive oil

4 shallots, finely chopped

2 carrots, finely diced

115 g/4 oz Puy lentils

450 ml/¾ pint red wine (optional)

Large handful of mixed dried seaweed flakes

Freshly ground black pepper

Mix all the marinade ingredients in a large shallow dish and turn the salmon in it. Cover and leave to marinate for about 1 hour, turning once or twice.

Cook the lentils: heat the oil in a heavy-based pan and sauté the shallots until translucent. Add the carrots and lentils and stir to coat well, then add the wine (if using) and seaweed. Season with pepper only. Bring to the boil, lower the heat, cover and simmer gently for about 30–40 minutes, until all the wine is absorbed and the lentils are tender.

Towards the end of this time, lightly oil a griddle pan and preheat it. Drain the salmon pieces from the marinade and pat dry. Arrange the salmon on the hot griddle pan at an angle, cook for 2 minutes and flip over to cook the other side for the same time. Turn again, this time also turning the salmon through 90 degrees so that the new set of sear marks will form an attractive crosshatch (or quadrillage) on the salmon. Cook for 2 minutes again, then flip over again to achieve the same on the other side. During this second set of searing, check with the tip of a sharp knife to see that the salmon is cooking all the way through; if not, extend the cooking by a minute or so on each – or just the final – side.

While the fish is cooking, bring the marinade to a simmer in a small pan to reduce by about half.

When ready, adjust the seasoning of the lentils and spoon them onto 4 warmed plates. Set a piece of salmon on top of each, spoon over some of the reduced marinade, then sprinkle with the sesame seeds and set a pat of chive butter on top of each.

ROAST NUT-COATED COD WITH A LEMON VINAIGRETTE DRESSING

P ★★　　E ★★★★　　A ★

This delicious dish goes very well with Champ or Colcannon mashed potatoes (see page 116). Both the miso broth and parsley provide good levels of plant oestrogens. The nuts, together with the linseed oil, contain an excellent mix of both Omega 3 and Omega 6 essential oils which are so good for combating premature ageing.

SERVES 4
PREPARATION: about 25 minutes
COOKING: about 20–35 minutes

1 tail end of cod, weighing about 800–900g/1¾–2lb

25g/1oz butter, plus more for greasing

Juice of 1 lemon, plus lemon slices for garnish

Freshly ground sea salt and black pepper

Small bunch of parsley, chopped, plus more whole sprigs to garnish

150ml/1¼ pint miso broth (see page 176) or fish stock (see page 177)

FOR THE COATING:

30g/1oz wholemeal breadcrumbs

15g/½oz ground almonds

30g/½oz flaked almonds

FOR THE LEMON VINAIGRETTE:

Juice and zest of 1 lemon

2 garlic cloves, finely chopped

Small bunch of flat-leaved parsley, finely chopped, plus more whole sprigs to garnish

115ml/4fl oz olive oil

2 tablespoons linseed oil

Buy the cod with the skin left on, but get the fishmonger to scale it for you, cut it open on one side and remove the bone.

Preheat the oven to 190°C/375°F/Gas 5 and butter an ovenproof dish. Rinse the cod carefully, including its cavity. Pat dry with paper towels. Put the fish in the prepared dish and sprinkle the lemon juice inside and outside the fish. Season lightly and sprinkle, again inside and out, with parsley. Dot the top with the butter and pour the stock around the base of the pan.

Roast for 20 minutes, basting regularly with the liquid in the pan.

After this time, mix together the coating ingredients and season well. Baste the fish and sprinkle the coating all over it. Return to the oven and cook for another 10–15 minutes, until the coating is nicely browned.

Meanwhile, mix together the ingredients for the lemon vinaigrette with seasoning to taste.

Serve the fish, garnished with lemon slices and parsley sprigs, accompanied by the vinaigrette.

FRITTEDDA PALERMITANA

P ★★　　E ★　　A ★

This traditional Sicilian artichoke, pea and broad bean stew is probably one of the nicest ways to use fresh young broad beans when they come into season. (See photograph opposite.)

Artichokes are interesting vegetables because they contain a substance called cynarin which is extremely beneficial to the liver. Cynarin improves liver function and has been said to stimulate liver cell regeneration. It is especially important that the liver is functioning optimally at the menopause so that the 'bad' oestrogens are converted into 'good' ones.

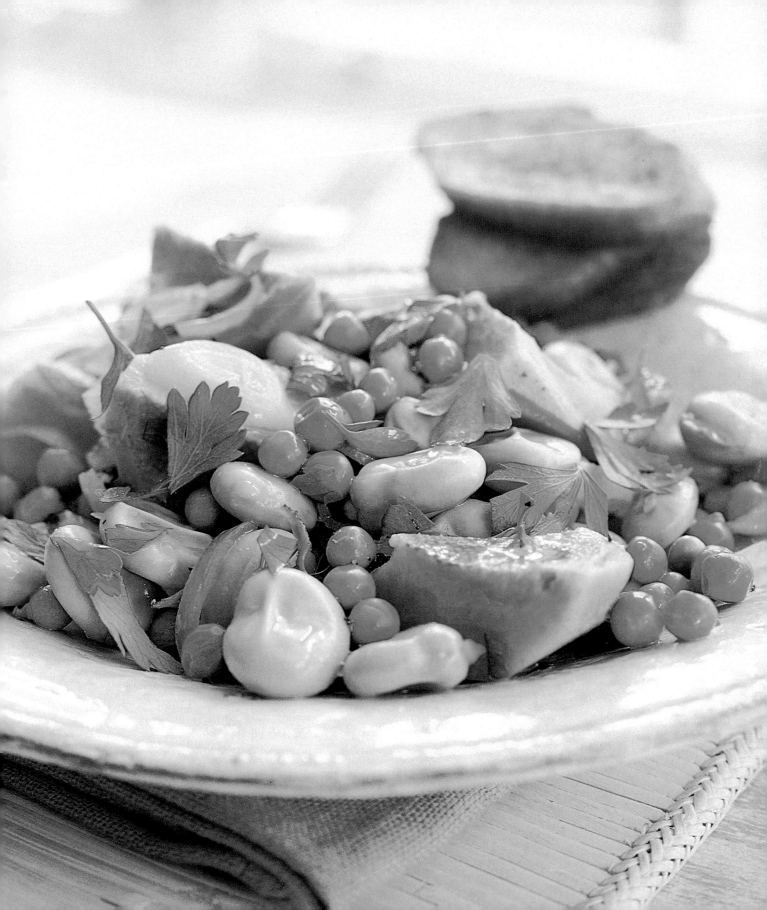

SERVES 6

PREPARATION: about 30 minutes

COOKING: about 35 minutes, plus cooling

6 large globe artichokes or 12–15 small young artichokes

Juice of ½ lemon

200 ml / 7 fl oz olive oil

300 g / 10½ oz large whole shallots

450 g / 1 lb shelled peas

450 g / 1 lb shelled fresh broad beans

Freshly ground sea salt and black pepper

100 ml / 3½ fl oz dry white wine

2 tablespoons chopped flat-leaved parsley, plus more whole leaves to garnish

Croûtes of good crusty bread fried in olive oil, to serve (optional)

First prepare the artichokes. For large artichokes, cut off the stalk and cut across to remove the top third of the leaves, remove any coarse outer leaves and halve lengthwise to remove the hairy choke inside, then cut each half again lengthwise into three pieces. Young artichokes (which have not developed their chokes) need only be trimmed of tough stalks and coarse outer leaves, then quartered. As they are prepared, drop them into a bowl of water acidulated with the lemon juice to prevent discoloration.

Heat the oil in a large heavy-based pan and fry the shallots gently until soft and translucent. Add the artichokes, peas and broad beans with seasoning to taste, followed by the wine and a ladleful of water and bring to the boil. Lower the heat to a gentle simmer, cover tightly and cook gently for about 20 minutes, or until the vegetables are tender. Stir from time to time and add a little more water if at any time it looks too dry. Add the chopped parsley for the last 5 minutes of cooking.

Serve hot, with croûtes of crusty bread fried in olive oil if you like, garnished with more whole parsley leaves.

VEGETABLE TEMPURA

P ★★ (with added tofu ★★★★)   E ★   A ★★

Tempura (see photograph opposite) uses a wonderful mix of vegetables and flavourings, but is definitely a dish to be kept for special occasions because it requires deep-frying. Frying oil at high temperatures can mean that the oil is damaged through the high temperature and creates free radicals. It is fine to treat yourself occasionally – after all, the dish does contain some wonderful ingredients which give health benefits. Moreover, the vinegar in the dipping sauce helps to break down the oils as the tempura is eaten.

Tofu can be cooked in the same way as the vegetables, and would make an easy and delicious introduction to the soya bean curd for those unfamiliar with it.

SERVES 6

PREPARATION: about 25 minutes

COOKING: 6–12 minutes

3 courgettes

1 large aubergine

1 head of broccoli

175 g / 6 oz large Portobello mushrooms

225 g / 8 oz asparagus

85 g / 3 oz sesame seeds

Olive oil for deep-frying

FOR THE DIPPING SAUCE:

150 ml / ¼ pint miso broth (see page 176) or vegetable stock (see page 177)

2 tablespoons soy sauce

2 tablespoons cider vinegar

2 tablespoons mirin (Japanese rice wine)

Freshly ground sea salt and black pepper

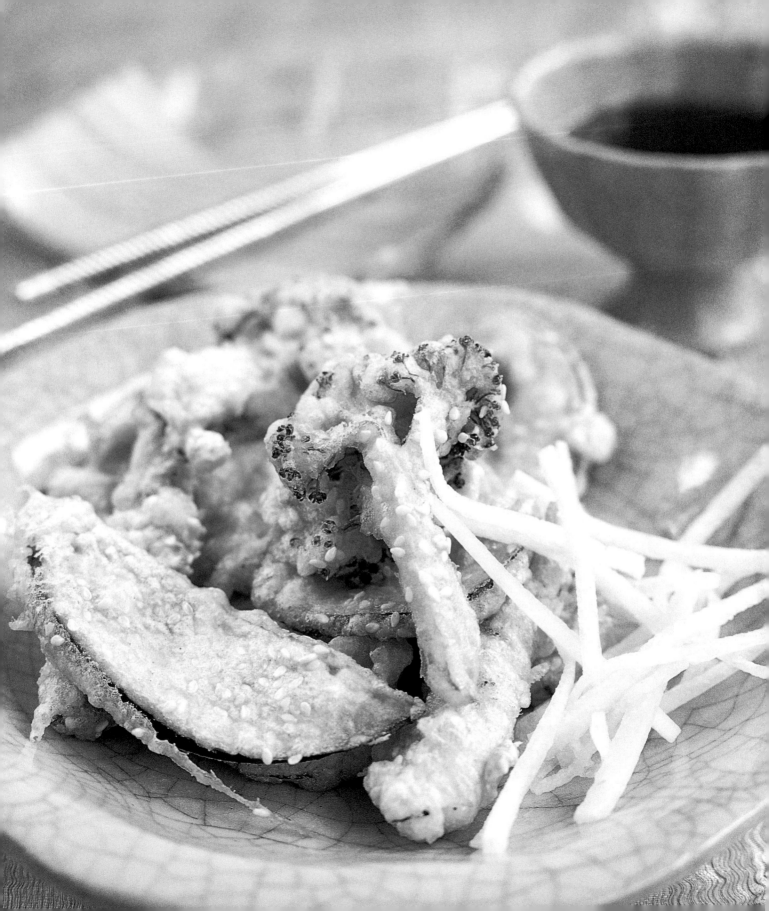

FOR THE TEMPURA BATTER:

1 large egg, plus 1 extra yolk

350 ml/12 fl oz iced water

175 g/6 oz plain flour, plus more for coating

1½ teaspoons baking powder

1 teaspoon salt

TO SERVE:

Fresh root ginger or Japanese pickled ginger, grated

Daikon (Japanese radish) or wasabi, freshly grated

Soy sauce

First make the dipping sauce: mix all the ingredients together in a small pan and place over a low heat to warm through.

Prepare the vegetables: slice the courgettes and aubergines across at an angle to give interestingly shaped slices. Separate the broccoli into bite-sized florets. Cut the mushrooms across into thickish slices. Trim the asparagus and cut in half if big. Pat all the vegetables thoroughly dry with paper towels.

When you are ready to fry, make the tempura batter: in a large bowl, beat the egg and extra yolk until just mixed. Stir in the iced water, then sift over the flour, baking powder and salt. Stir until just combined – do not over-mix (there should still be visible flecks of flour) or the batter will be heavy.

Preheat a low oven to 190°C/375°F/Gas 5 and heat the oil for deep-frying very hot, so that a stale bread cube will brown in it in 40 seconds.

To cook the vegetables, toss the pieces one at a time in flour and then dip them in the batter to coat completely, shake off any excess and sprinkle with sesame seeds. Drop them into the hot oil for 2–3 minutes, until golden, then remove with a slotted spoon and drain on paper towels. You will probably have to work in batches (never overcrowd the pan when deep-frying as this lowers the cooking temperature too much and the batter or food goes soggy): keep the cooked pieces hot in the warm oven with the door open until all are cooked.

Serve hot with the dipping sauce and accompaniments.

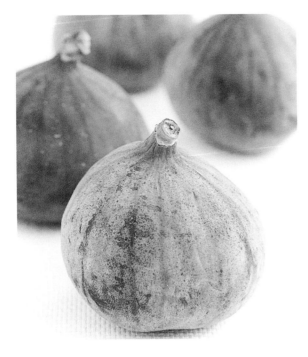

Hot
and cold
desserts

FRUIT KEBABS

P ★★★   E ★   A ★★★★

This is an unusual and rewarding way to serve fruit: not only is it pretty, but the grilling makes the fruit extra fragrant and sweet. The soya yoghurt supplies phytoestrogens and the almonds are full of essential oils. The fruit itself offers an excellent variety of different kinds of powerful antioxidants – so important for combating free radicals and preventing premature ageing.

SERVES 4

PREPARATION: about 30 minutes

COOKING: 3–4 minutes

900g/2lb assorted firm fruit such as apples, pears, plums, grapes, cherries, persimmon, figs, peaches, nectarines, strawberries, apricot, mango, papaya

Juice of 1–2 lemons

40g/1½oz flaked almonds, plus more to garnish

Yoghurt, preferably soya yoghurt, to serve

FOR THE GINGER AND CINNAMON BUTTER:

5-cm/2-in piece of root ginger

55g/2oz softened unsalted butter

2 tablespoons maple syrup

1 teaspoon ground cinnamon

Soak 8 small wooden skewers in water, so they won't burn during cooking. Preheat a hot grill or light a barbecue.

As appropriate, core, deseed and stone the fruit, leaving smaller fruit whole and cutting the larger fruit into large bite-sized chunks. Leave edible skins on as they will help hold the cooking fruit together. As you work, sprinkle the cut fruit with lemon juice to prevent discoloration.

Arrange the prepared fruit attractively on the skewers.

Make the ginger cinnamon butter: squeeze the juice from the ginger (use a garlic press or piece of muslin) into a small bowl, add the remaining ingredients and mash together.

Using a pastry brush, coat the fruit on the skewers liberally with the butter, then sprinkle with the almonds. Sprinkle any remaining nuts and butter in the bottom of a grill pan, if grilling.

Grill or barbecue the kebabs for about 1½–2 minutes on each side, basting them fairly constantly with more of the ginger cinnamon butter or the pan juices.

Serve immediately, sprinkled with any remaining butter or pan juices and almonds, accompanied by yoghurt.

MINTED FRUIT SALAD

P ★★★★   E ★★★★   A ★★★★★

This salad (see photograph opposite) also makes a perfect first course on a warm summer's day. Obviously, the mix of fruit used in the salad can be adjusted according to season.

This particular combination of pretty berries and firm-fleshed fruit gives the dish excellent anti-ageing and anti-cancer benefits. The soya yoghurt supplies phytoestrogens, which the linseeds top up if sprinkled in. Linseeds also contain both Omega 3 and Omega 6 essential fatty acids. The addition of mint jazzes up the salad wonderfully, lending it a fresh, leafy tang without destroying the subtle flavours of the individual fruit. A real treat.

SERVES 6–8

PREPARATION: about 15 minutes, plus chilling

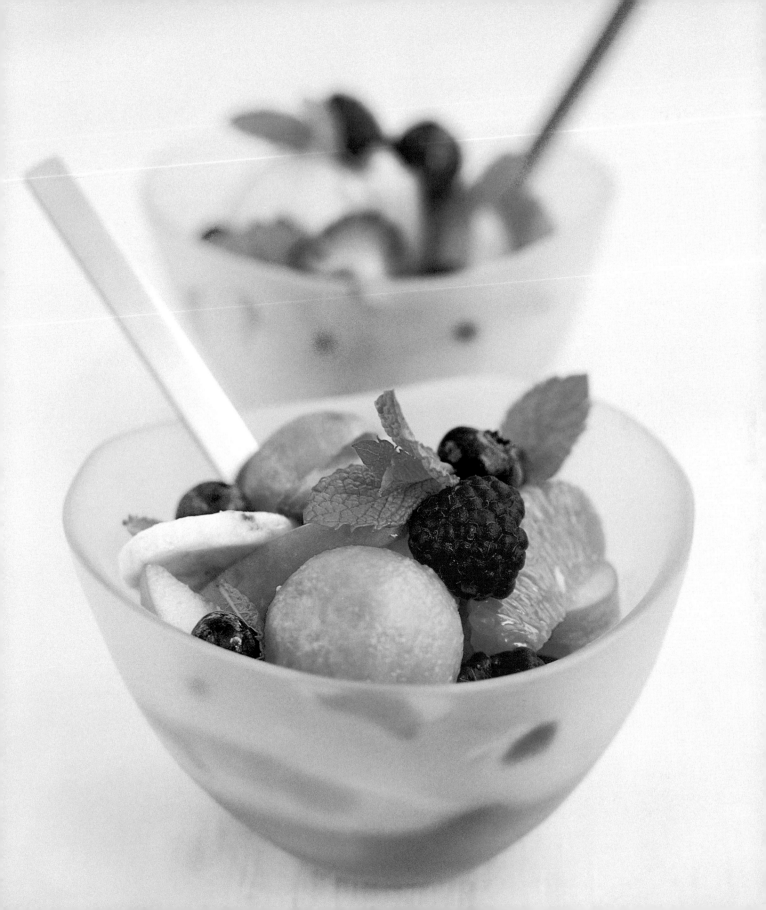

Juice of 1 lemon

5 tablespoons honey

2 tablespoons fresh mint leaves, finely chopped, plus more whole leaves to decorate

2 oranges

225 g / 8 oz seedless black grapes

2 ripe pears

2 ripe firm-fleshed apples

2 bananas

1 small ripe melon

225 g / 8 oz mixed berry fruit in season, such as strawberries, raspberries, blueberries

Soya yoghurt or cream, to serve

Mix the lemon juice, honey and chopped mint in the bottom of a large bowl. As you prepare the fruit, stir it into this mixture, trying to add any juices to the bowl. Peel the oranges and then cut down into each segment to release the flesh from its envelope of skin; halve the grapes, if large; halve and core the unpeeled pears and apples and cut into bite-sized chunks; peel and slice the bananas; halve and deseed the melon and scoop out the flesh using a melon baller or sharp-edged teaspoon. Chill for at least an hour.

Just before serving, mix in the berry fruit and decorate with sprigs of mint. Serve with soya yoghurt or cream.

Variation: to boost the phytoestrogen content, you could sprinkle a couple of tablespoons of linseeds into the salad with the berry fruit and or add some freshly squeezed juice from a lump of root ginger (chop finely and squeeze in a piece of muslin or in a garlic press).

STUFFED PEARS IN RED WINE

P ★★★   E ★   A ★★★

Pears have such a delicate flavour and are such an elegant shape that they give any dessert a touch of class. Their marriage with red wine here delivers high amounts of antioxidants – so good for preventing premature ageing – and the soya yoghurt provides phytoestrogens.

SERVES 4

PREPARATION: 20 minutes, plus 2 hours' soaking

COOKING: about 20 minutes

2 tablespoons sultanas

1 tablespoon cider vinegar

1 lemon

4 large firm pears

300 ml / ½ pint red wine

3 tablespoons honey

1 cinnamon stick

1 level tablespoon black peppercorns

Soya yoghurt, to serve

At least 2 hours before you intend to cook the pears, put the sultanas in a small bowl and pour over the vinegar and the juice of half the lemon. Toss to mix well.

Peel the pears and halve them carefully lengthwise, leaving the stalks attached to one half. Scoop out the cores.

Pour the red wine into a saucepan just big enough to hold the pear halves snugly. Heat gently and stir in the honey, cinnamon, peppercorns and 3 tablespoons of the remaining lemon juice.

When the honey has dissolved, put the pears in the liquid and spoon some over their tops. Cover and poach at the gentlest possible simmer for

15–20 minutes, turning the pears from time to time and spooning liquid over them, until the pears are translucent and tender but still quite firm.

Remove the pears to a serving dish and strain the liquid. When the pears are cool enough to handle, stuff the cavities of 4 of the pear halves with a mounded spoonful of the macerated sultanas. Reassemble with the other matching pear half and wrap tightly in greaseproof paper. Put the pear packages and liquid to chill in the fridge for at least 2–3 hours.

To serve, unwrap the packages and spoon over some of the reserved poaching liquid. Serve with some yoghurt flavoured with a couple of spoonfuls of the poaching liquid.

SUMMER PUDDING WITH ELDERFLOWER YOGHURT

P ★★★   E ★   A ★★★★

Another very simple dessert, this is full of natural sweetness and goodness. The elderflower tea is effective as an anti-inflammatory for the joints, the soya yoghurt contains plenty of plant hormones and all the berries are an excellent store of antioxidants.

SERVES 6–8
PREPARATION: about 20 minutes
COOKING: 3–4 minutes, plus several hours' chilling

6–8 thick slices of day-old wholemeal bread
800g/1¾lb mixed fruits, including a good proportion of raspberries and redcurrants and some of the following: strawberries, blueberries, stoned cherries, blackberries or loganberries
4–5 tablespoons runny honey

FOR THE ELDERFLOWER YOGHURT:
1 sachet (1 heaped tablespoon) of elderflower tea
250ml/9floz soya yoghurt
2 tablespoons runny honey

Remove the crusts from the bread and use most of the slices to line the bottom and sides of a 850-ml/½-pint pudding basin, cutting the bread to get a good fit if necessary.

Put all the fruit in a large heavy-based pan and drizzle over the honey. Put over a very low heat. Cook for 3–4 minutes only, stirring carefully from time to time until the juices just begin to run but the fruit is not losing any of its shape.

Remove the pan from the heat and spoon the fruit and juices into the lined pudding basin, reserving 2–3 tablespoons of the juices in a small jug. Cover the pudding with more pieces of bread cut to fit and place a small plate with a diameter just less than that of the rim of the basin on top of the pudding. Weight this down with a couple of tins. Chill for 3–4 hours, or preferably overnight.

Make the elderflower yoghurt: put the elderflower tea in a heatproof bowl and pour 2 tablespoons of boiling water over it. Leave to steep for about 15 minutes.

Put the yoghurt in another bowl, strain in the elderflower infusion and stir in the honey. Chill until you want to serve.

When ready to serve, remove the weights and plate and turn the pudding out on a serving plate. Trickle over the reserved juices, taking care to cover any patches of the bread crust which are still pale. Serve cut in wedges, with some of the elderflower yoghurt.

MIXED BERRY SOUFFLÉ OMELETTE

P ★★★   E ★★   A ★★★★

Eggs are full of nutrients and, even though they are high in cholesterol, studies have shown that they do not increase cholesterol levels in the body. The tofu cream in this omelette (see photograph, page 2) gives excellent phyto-estrogen levels and the berries are a great source of anti-ageing and anti-cancer antioxidants.

You could also make 4 individual soufflé omelettes, using a small crêpe or blini pan. You would, however, have to serve them as they were cooked. For entertaining, you could perhaps sprinkle the omelette with a very little icing sugar to make it look more attractive.

SERVES 4–6
PREPARATION: about 15 minutes
COOKING: about 15 minutes

3 tablespoons honey
Pinch of ground cinnamon
5 tablespoons crème fraîche or tofu cream
6 large eggs
1 tablespoon lemon juice
Freshly ground black pepper
225 g/8 oz mixed berry fruit such as raspberries, blueberries and strawberries
25 g/1 oz butter

In a large bowl, mix half the honey and the cinnamon into the crème fraîche or tofu cream. Separate the eggs, beat the yolks lightly and mix into the cream mixture.

In a small bowl, mix the remaining honey and the lemon juice with a grinding of black pepper. When they are well mixed, add the berries and toss to coat them well.

In another (very clean and dry) large bowl, beat the egg whites until standing in stiff peaks. Take 2 or 3 large spoonfuls of this and add to the cream mixture. Mix well to loosen the mixture. Then add the remaining egg whites and fold in lightly but thoroughly, using the side of a large metal spoon.

Put a flameproof serving dish in to warm (but don't let it get too hot) and preheat a fairly hot grill. Melt the butter in a large heavy frying pan over a moderate heat.

When the butter is just on the point of turning colour, add the cream mixture and cook over a low to moderate heat until the edges start to puff. Shake the pan from time to time. As soon as the omelette starts to move freely around in the pan, indicating the bottom has set, spoon the berries over one half of the omelette, making sure they go right out to the edge so they can be glimpsed when the omelette is folded. Fold the other side of the omelette over the fruit and slide it out onto the warmed serving dish.

Place under the grill and cook until well risen, then serve at once, cutting into wedges at the table.

FRUIT TART

P ★★   E ★★★   A ★★★

If you are short of time you can buy ready-made wholemeal pastry cases in health food shops. Of course, they are never as good as the homemade variety but the ingredients are healthy. However, bought pastry does not contain soya flour, which this recipe does. (See photograph opposite.)

Essential oils are present in the nuts and sesame seeds and good levels of antioxidants in the fruit.

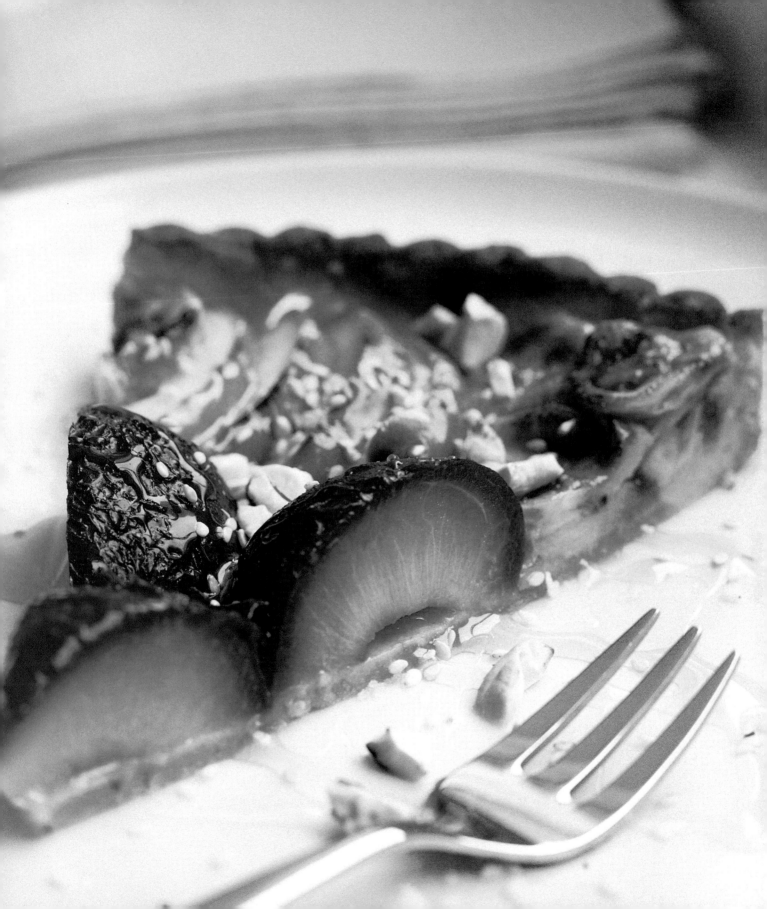

SERVES 6–8

PREPARATION: about 1 hour

COOKING: 25–30 minutes

225 g / 8 oz plums, halved and stoned

3–4 firm dessert apples, halved, cored and sliced

2–3 large ripe bananas, peeled and sliced

FOR THE PASTRY:

150 g / 5 oz plain, preferably wholemeal, flour

25 g / 1 oz soya flour

Large pinch of freshly ground salt

175 g / 6 oz soft unsalted butter, diced small

2 egg yolks

2 tablespoons honey

Zest of 1 small orange, grated

FOR THE GLAZE:

4 tablespoons maple syrup

15 g / ½ oz butter

1 cup cashew nuts or macadamia nuts, lightly toasted and coarsely chopped

2 tablespoons sesame seeds, lightly toasted

Make the pastry: sift the flours and salt into a large bowl, make a well in the centre and add the diced butter. Mix in lightly. In a small bowl, beat the egg yolks lightly with the honey and 3 tablespoons of water. Add this to the flour mixture with the orange zest. Work the ingredients together with the finger-tips until it coheres (you may need a very little more water). Roll into a ball and knead briefly and lightly.

Roll out on a lightly floured surface and use to line a 25-cm / 10-in shallow tart pan. Leave to rest in the refrigerator for a short while. Preheat the oven to 190°C/375°F/Gas 5.

Arrange the fruit decoratively on the tart base: concentric circles with the plum halves, cut side down, in the centre, the apple around them and the bananas around the outside look good. Bake for 25–30 minutes until the pastry edges are a deep colour and the fruit is tender when pierced.

Meanwhile make the glaze by mixing the maple syrup and butter in a heavy-based pan. As soon as it comes to the boil, stop stirring and allow it to simmer until it starts to thicken. Remove from the heat and dip the base of the pan in cold water to stop the cooking process. Keep warm.

When the tart comes out of the oven, pour the glaze uniformly over the top and sprinkle with the nuts and seeds. Serve warm.

APRICOT TOFU ICE-CREAM

P ★ ★ ★ ★   E ★   A ★ ★ ★ ★

Apricots are an excellent source of beta-carotene, the most important antioxidant. They also contain potassium, which helps reduce high blood pressure and water retention. The tofu supplies a high degree of plant hormones.

SERVES 6

PREPARATION: about 10 minutes

COOKING: 3–4 minutes, plus 1 hour's freezing

400 ml / 14 fl oz apple juice

2 tablespoons agar agar seaweed

85 g / 3 oz dried apricots, stewed, drained and cooled

450 g / 1 lb soft tofu

Pour the apple juice into a saucepan and sprinkle over the agar agar. Bring to a simmer and cook gently until the agar agar is dissolved, a few minutes.

Pour into a blender or food processor and add the apricots and tofu. Blend until smooth.

Freeze until firm but not solid, 1 hour. Leave to soften in the fridge for 15 minutes before serving.

BANANA CREAM PIE

P ★★★★   E ★   A ★

This seems a wicked pie but does not have the usual cream and eggs. The filling is set with agar, a seaweed which comes in white flakes and contains a number of excellent nutrients including iodine.

SERVES 4–6
PREPARATION: about 30 minutes, plus cooling
COOKING: about 5 minutes, plus cooling and chilling

FOR THE CRUST:
3 tablespoons corn oil
4 tablespoons maple syrup
175 g/6 oz wholemeal flour

FOR THE FILLING:
1 tablespoon arrowroot
600 ml/1 pint soya milk
3 tablespoons agar agar seaweed
3 tablespoons maple syrup
Zest of 1 orange
½ teaspoon vanilla extract
2 ripe bananas, very thinly sliced

Preheat the oven to 180°C/350°F/Gas 4.

First make the crust: mix the oil and syrup in a blender or food processor and pour into a mixing bowl. Mix in the flour and rub in with the fingertips until fully mixed and a crumbly consistency. Compact the mixture into the base and up the sides of a 23-cm/9-in pie dish. Allow to cool.

Make the filling: in a small bowl, mix the arrowroot with 2 tablespoons of the soya milk and set aside. Put the remaining soya milk, agar agar, maple syrup and orange zest in a saucepan, bring to a simmer and cook gently for 3 minutes. Add the arrowroot solution and continue to cook, stirring constantly, until thick. Remove from the heat.

Stir in the vanilla followed by the banana slices. Pour the mixture into the cooled crust and chill for 1 hour, or until set.

TOFU CHEESECAKE

P ★★★★   E ★   A ★

This dish makes a change from a dairy cheesecake and, of course, delivers the health benefits of the phytoestrogens in the tofu. The sesame seed paste (tahini) gives an excellent amount of calcium.

SERVES 4–6
PREPARATION: about 5 minutes, plus making the crust
COOKING: 35–40 minutes, plus cooling

1 pie crust (see Banana Cream Pie, adjacent)

FOR THE FILLING:
Four 225-g/8-oz packs of soft tofu
4–8 tablespoons maple syrup, to taste
6 tablespoons tahini
1 teaspoon vanilla essence
2 teaspoons lemon juice
Pinch of freshly ground sea salt

Preheat the oven to 180°C/350°F/Gas 4.

Make the filling: crumble the tofu into a blender or food processor. Add the remaining ingredients and blend until smooth.

Pour into the pie crust and bake for 35–40 minutes, until the pastry is a light golden brown. Allow to cool before serving.

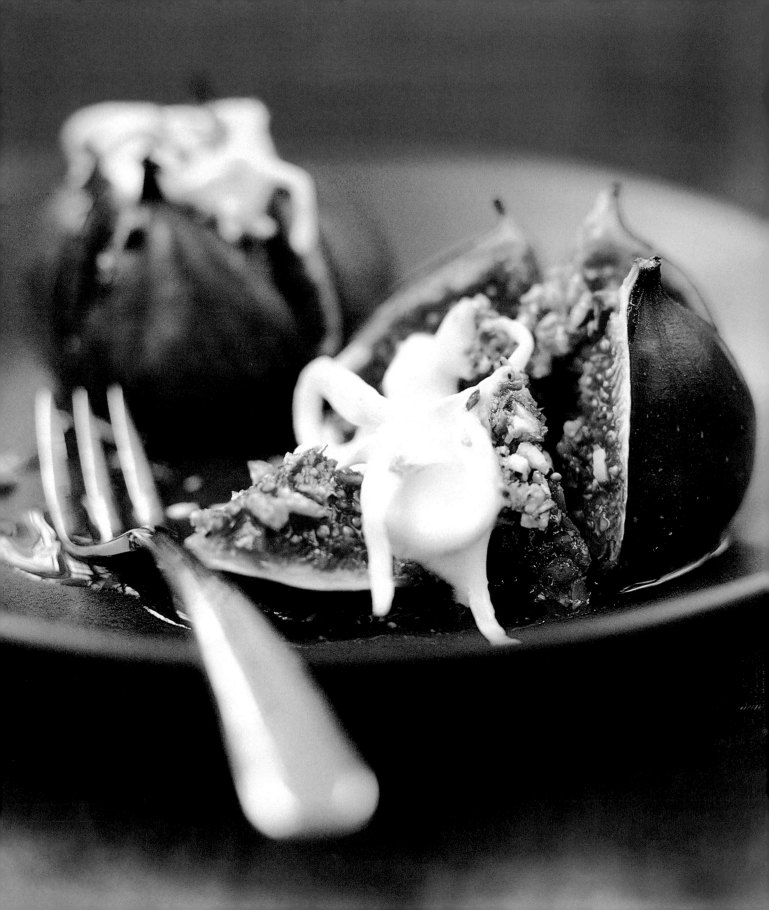

BAKED FIGS

P ★★★   E ★★   A ★

Figs contain pectin, a soluble fibre, which is good for the bowels and helps lower cholesterol levels. They also contain an enzyme called ficin, which aids digestion, and are a good source of calcium. The soya yoghurt provides the phyto-estrogens in this dessert and the pistachio nuts bring essential oils. (See photograph opposite.)

SERVES 6
PREPARATION: 15 minutes
COOKING: about 15 minutes, plus cooling

18 ripe figs
85 g/3 oz pistachio nuts, coarsely chopped, reserving
a few for decoration
4 tablespoons honey
Zest of 1 large orange, grated
175 ml/6 fl oz soya yoghurt

Preheat the oven to 200°C/400°F/Gas 6.

Shave off a thin sliver from the fat end of each fig so they will sit upright without falling over. Cut a cross in the top end of each fig, to about halfway down. Ease the figs open, squeezing the bottom halves if necessary.

Mix together the chopped pistachios and honey. Spoon this mixture into the figs and bake for about 15 minutes. Allow to cool slightly.

In a small bowl, mix the orange zest into the yoghurt. Spoon this into the figs and decorate with the reserved pistachios before serving warm.

MIXED BERRY FOOL

P ★★★★   E ★   A ★★★★★

Mixed berries contain proanthocyanidins, which are excellent antioxidants. They are useful in preventing osteoporosis since they stop the destruction of collagen and strengthen the collagen matrix. With their powerful antioxidant properties, they also play a major part in the prevention of heart disease and strokes. This tangy fool is also rich in phytoestrogens from the tofu.

SERVES 4
PREPARATION: about 10 minutes, plus chilling

450 g/1 lb mixed berries of the season
225 g/8 oz soft tofu, chilled
Dash of vanilla extract
Maple syrup to taste
A little soya milk, chilled

Reserving a few of each type of berry for decoration, put all the ingredients except the soya milk in a blender or food processor. Process well until smooth.

If too thick, let down with a little soya milk if necessary to give a good consistency (it should be like cream whipped to soft peaks).

Spoon into clear glasses and decorate with the reserved berries. Chill briefly before serving.

Variation: if you have the time, purée half the berries on their own with some maple syrup to taste and build up layers of fool and purée in the glasses for a really attractive effect.

ATHOLL BROSE

P ★★★★   E ★   A ★

This aristocratic pudding is said to have been invented by and named after a Duke of Atholl. Oats are excellent for the heart because they naturally contain oat bran and are also a source of phytoestrogens. This dish is a perfect vehicle for using them in something other than a breakfast cereal – which makes a change. The soya cream supplies extra phytoestrogens. Use the whisky for very special occasions only.

SERVES 4
PREPARATION: about 5 minutes, plus chilling

50g/2oz fine oatmeal, toasted
4 tablespoons good honey, preferably heather honey, plus more to serve
300ml/½ pint soya cream
6 tablespoons Scotch whisky (optional)

Mix the oatmeal and honey into the soya cream and chill well.

Stir in the whisky (if using) just before serving, topped with another spoonful of the honey.

CLAFOUTIS

P ★★★   E ★   A ★★★

This is marvellously simple to make, and quite delicious as well as healthy. (See photograph opposite.) The soya milk gives a good supply of plant hormones and the cherries contain useful antioxidants.

SERVES 6
PREPARATION: about 15 minutes
COOKING: 35–40 minutes

25g/1oz butter
100g/3½oz flour
½ teaspoon freshly ground sea salt
300ml/½ pint soya milk
4 eggs
3 tablespoons honey
100ml/3½floz kirsch
450g/1lb ripe tart black cherries

Preheat the oven to 180°C/350°F/Gas 4 and put a shallow baking dish containing the butter in the oven.

In a large bowl, mix the flour, salt, milk, eggs, honey and kirsch to a smooth batter.

When the oven is at the right temperature, take out the hot tin and tilt it at all angles to coat it well with the melted butter. Pour in the batter, then sprinkle the cherries into the batter and return to the oven for about 35–40 minutes, until well puffed-up and coloured.

Serve warm, and don't worry that it sinks as it cools – this is normal.

Variation: you can also make this dessert using stoned black cherries from a tin – make sure you drain them first.

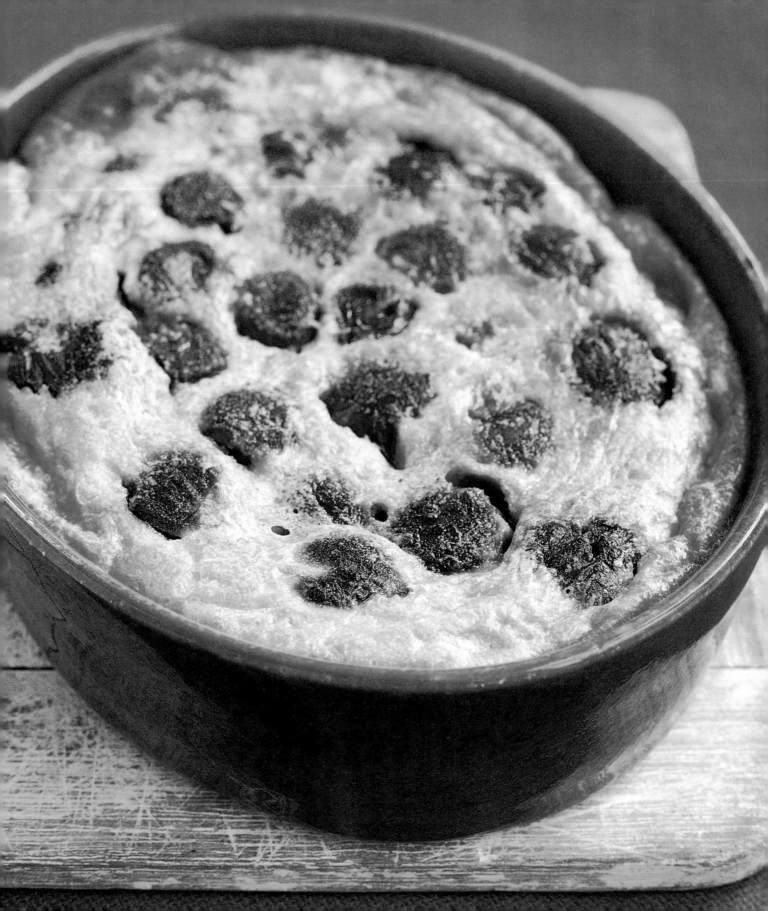

STRAWBERRY SHORTCAKE

P ★★★★   E ★★   A ★★★

The queen of the summer fruits, the strawberry is also an excellent source of antioxidants. It contains more vitamin C than any other berry so it is very good for the immune system and also helps to produce collagen for skin and bone health. The shortcake's phytoestrogen content – in the soya flour and milk as well as the tofu cream – is very high. (See photograph, page 19.)

SERVES 8

PREPARATION: about 45 minutes, plus 2 hours' macerating

COOKING: 10–12 minutes

175 g/6 oz strawberries, halved or thickly sliced (depending on size)

3 tablespoons maple syrup

Squeeze of lemon juice

FOR THE SHORTCAKE DOUGH:

150 g/5 oz wholemeal flour

225 g/8 oz plain flour, plus more for dusting

2 heaped tablespoons soya flour

1 tablespoon baking powder

Pinch of freshly ground salt

85 g/3 oz cold unsalted butter, diced, plus more for glazing

3 tablespoons honey, plus more for glazing

150 ml/¼ pint soya milk

FOR THE FILLING:

285 g/10 oz silken tofu

2 tablespoons honey

1 uncoated orange, finely grated

2 tablespoons brandy

2 tablespoons vanilla essence

In a bowl, gently toss the strawberry slices in the maple syrup and lemon juice. Set aside to macerate for at least 2 hours, tossing from time to time.

Towards the end of this time, make the shortcakes: preheat the oven to 230°C/450°F/Gas 8. Sift the flours, baking powder and salt into a large bowl. Add the butter and, using your fingers, rub into the flour until the mixture resembles coarse crumbs. Add the honey and all but a spoonful or two of the soya milk. Stir gently until a dough forms; if it is too thick (it should be soft but not too sloppy), add the remaining milk.

With floured hands and on a floured surface, roll it into a ball and knead for about 30 seconds. Then pat out to a round about 2 cm/¾ in thick. Using a 7-cm/2¾-in pastry cutter, cut out rounds, re-rolling as necessary to get 8 rounds. Arrange on a baking sheet, spaced well apart.

In a pan melt a little butter, then mix in some honey and brush the tops of the rounds as a glaze. Bake for about 10–12 minutes until well risen and golden. Transfer to a wire rack to cool until they are no longer hot, but warm.

Make the filling: in a blender or food processor, blend together all the ingredients until smooth and slightly aerated.

Split each of the warm shortcakes across into two halves and spread the two bottom halves with a little of the filling. Arrange a thick layer of strawberry slices on top of each and then cover generously with filling. Put the shortcake top halves in place on top, cover with another thick layer of filling, strawberry slices and more filling if there is any left. Arrange any remaining strawberry slices decoratively around the shortcakes, pour the strawberry juices around the plates and serve immediately.

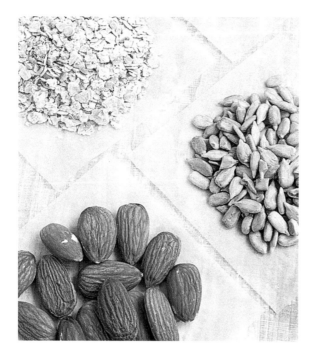

Breads,
cakes
and
biscuits

DELUXE FLAPJACKS

P ★★★★   E ★★★★   A ★

Blissfully quick to make, flapjacks make a perfect tea-time or mid-morning treat and are full of nutritious ingredients. Phytoestrogens are provided by the seeds and oats and good quantities of essential oils by the seeds and almonds. The apricots contain beta-carotene, an excellent antioxidant.

MAKES about 20
PREPARATION: about 20 minutes
COOKING: 15–20 minutes, plus cooling

125g/4½oz butter, plus more for greasing
6 tablespoons apple concentrate
1 tablespoon linseeds
1 tablespoon sunflower seeds
1 tablespoon sesame seeds
½ teaspoon ground cinnamon
½ teaspoon ground ginger
225g/8oz rolled oats
1 tablespoon flaked almonds
40g/1½oz seedless raisins, chopped
40g/1½oz no-need-to-soak dried apricots, chopped

Preheat the oven to 180°C/350°F/Gas 4 and butter a Swiss roll tin.

In a small pan over a low heat, melt the butter with the apple concentrate, seeds and spices. Stir in the oats, nuts and fruit, and mix well.

Spread the mixture about 5–10mm/¼-1.2in thick in the prepared tin and bake for about 15–20 minutes, until golden.

Allow to cool slightly and then mark into rectangles with a knife and break into pieces. Allow to cool completely.

CHOCOLATE BROWNIES

P ★★★   E ★★   A ★

These brownies (see photograph opposite) are for a special treat but are still much healthier than shop-bought ones. The soya and wholemeal flours give phytoestrogens and the nuts essential oils. As the nuts are cooked inside the brownies, the quality of the oils is somewhat protected.

MAKES about 30
PREPARATION: about 20 minutes
COOKING: 25 minutes, plus cooling

115g/4oz butter, plus more for greasing
55g/2oz 100 per cent cocoa powder, sifted
Large pinch of freshly ground salt
1 teaspoon baking powder
3 eggs (at room temperature), beaten
350ml/12floz date or maple syrup
2 teaspoons vanilla extract
115g/4oz wholemeal flour, sifted
2 heaped tablespoons soya flour, sifted
85g/3oz pecan nuts, coarsely chopped
85g/3oz dates, coarsely chopped

Preheat the oven to 180°C/350°F/Gas 4 and butter a 23×30-cm/9×12-in cake pan.

In a large mixing bowl, cream together the butter and cocoa powder until smooth. Beat in the salt and baking powder, followed by the eggs a little at a time, and continue to beat until well creamed. Add the date or maple syrup and vanilla and combine quickly with a few stirs of the spoon.

While this mixture is still streaky, fold in the flours and then, while that is still streaky, gently stir in the nuts and dates. Spoon into the prepared pan.

Bake for 25 minutes and leave to cool in the tin. Turn out and cut into bars to serve.

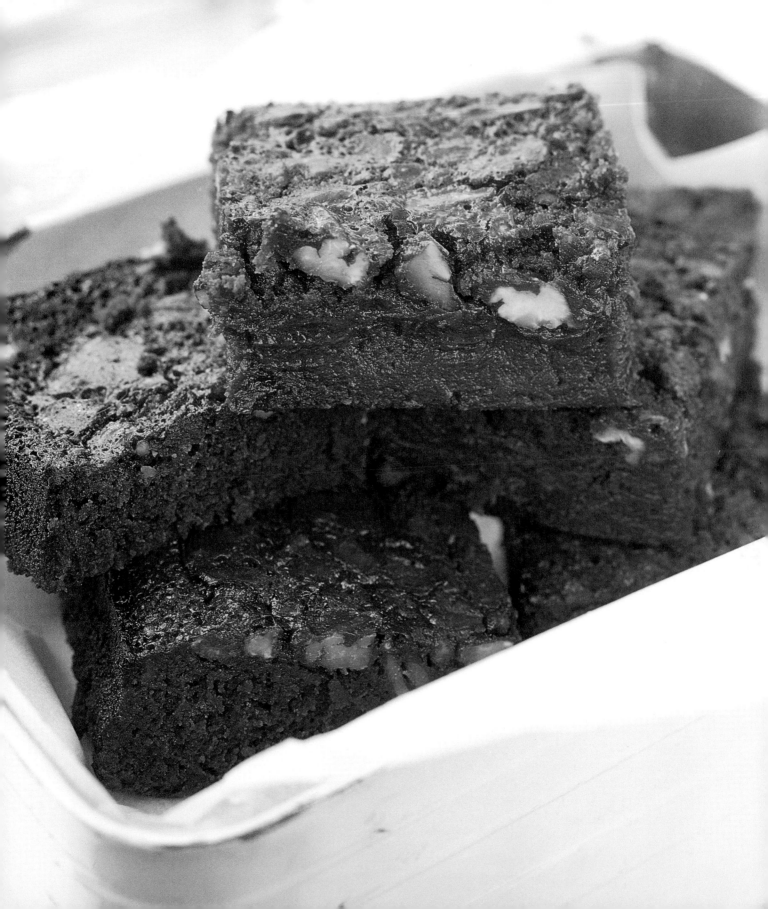

BANANA BREAD

P ★ ★ ★   E ★   A ★

Banana bread has no need for added sugar as it is naturally sweet. The addition of apricots and nuts makes this recipe especially delicious. Bananas are an excellent fruit as they are high in both potassium (useful with water retention) and pectin, which is a soluble fibre that can help lower cholesterol. Plant oestrogens are present in the soya and wholemeal flours.

MAKES 1 medium loaf
PREPARATION: about 20 minutes
COOKING: about 1 hour, plus cooling

Butter or olive oil for greasing
55 g/2 oz slightly salted butter
125 ml/4½ fl oz date syrup
Zest of 1 lemon, finely grated
2 eggs, lightly beaten
3 large ripe (or overripe) bananas, mashed
225 g/8 oz wholemeal self-raising flour
2 tablespoons soya flour
55 g/2 oz pecan nuts or walnuts, chopped
55 g/2 oz dried apricots, chopped

Preheat the oven to 190°C/375°F/Gas 5 and grease a large loaf tin. In a large mixing bowl, cream the butter with the syrup and lemon zest, then beat in the eggs followed by the banana purée. Sift in one-third of the mixed flours and beat until smooth, then add the rest of the flours in the same way. Fold in the nuts and fruit. Pour and spoon into the loaf tin. Level the top.

    Bake for about 1 hour, until golden in colour and springy to the touch. Turn out of the tin and allow to cool on a wire rack.

NUTTY GINGERBREAD

P ★ ★ ★ ★   E ★ ★   A ★

The soya milk and flour give phytoestrogens and the nuts essential oils. Ginger is beneficial for the circulation. (See photograph opposite.)

MAKES about 16 small squares
PREPARATION: about 20 minutes, plus cooling
COOKING: 30–40 minutes, plus cooling

Butter or olive oil for greasing
85 g/3 oz butter
4 tablespoons soya milk
2 eggs
200 ml/7 fl oz date syrup
150 g/5 oz wholemeal self-raising flour
25 g/1 oz soya flour
1 teaspoon bicarbonate of soda
1 tablespoon ground ginger
1 teaspoon ground cinnamon
½ teaspoon ground mixed spice
25 g/1 oz almonds, chopped
25 g/1 oz walnuts, chopped

Preheat the oven to 180°C/350°F/Gas 4 and grease a 23-cm/9-in square cake tin. Line it with baking paper and grease that too. Heat the milk and melt the 85 g/3 oz butter in it, then let cool to lukewarm. Whisk in the egg and date syrup until combined.

    Sift the flours, bicarbonate of soda and spices into a large bowl. Stir in the chopped nuts. Make a well in the centre. Pour the milk mixture into the well and stir together until a smooth batter forms.

    Pour into the tin and smooth the top. Bake for 30–40 minutes, until a skewer inserted comes out dry. Allow to cool on a wire rack. Turn out of the tin, remove the paper and cut into squares to serve.

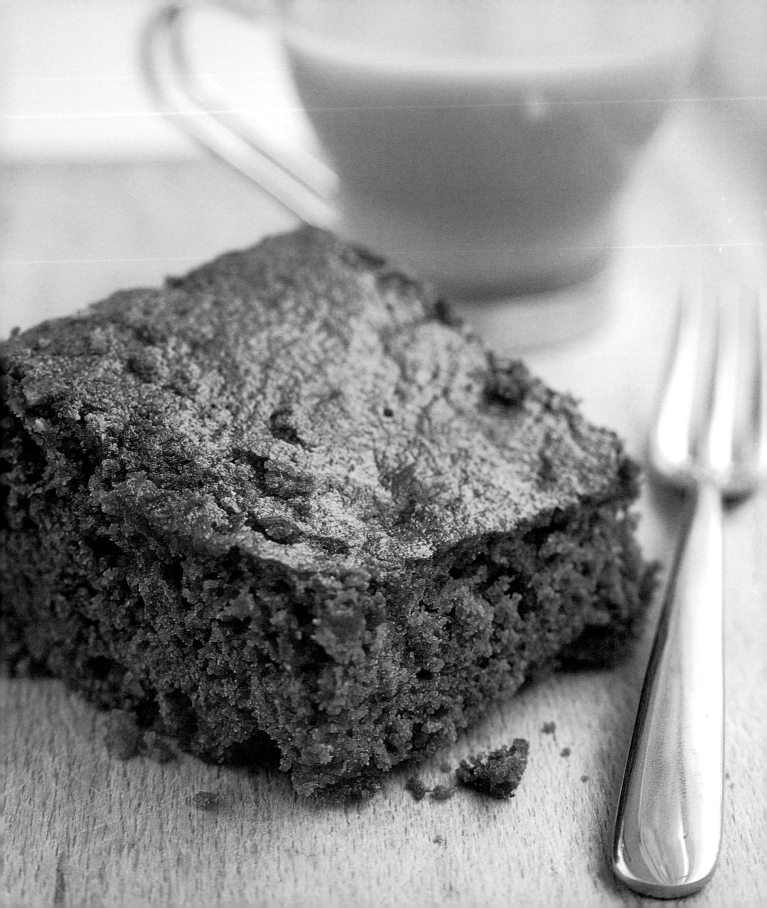

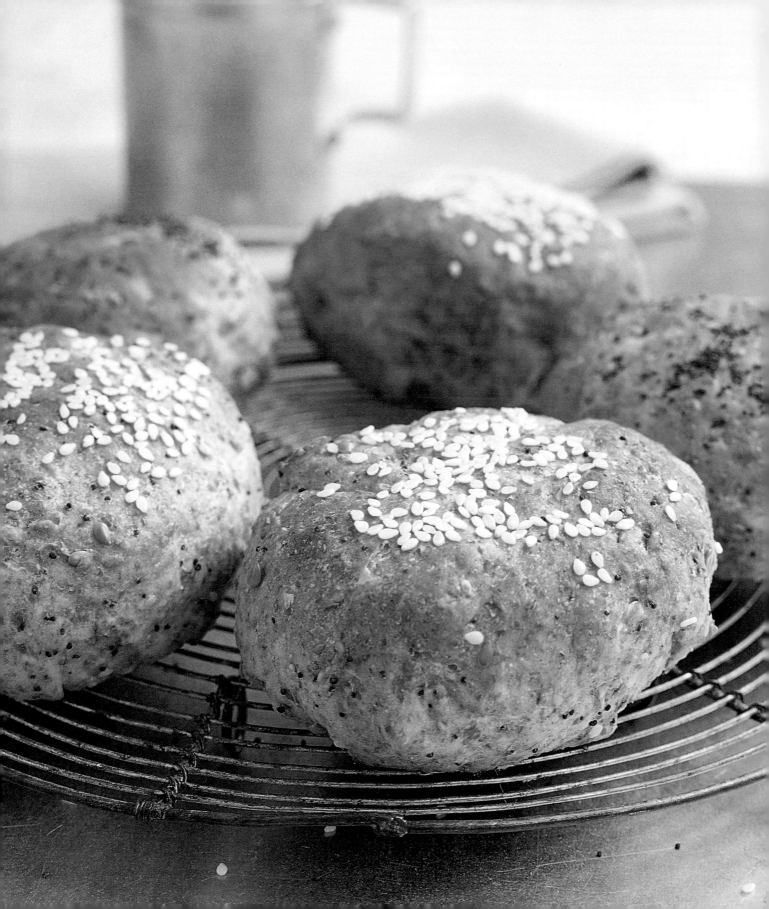

SEED ROLLS

P ★★★★   E ★★★   A ★

There are lots of plant oestrogens in these rolls (see photograph opposite), particularly from the linseeds but also from the other seeds and soya milk. Essential oils are supplied by the seeds.

MAKES about 8

PREPARATION: about 30 minutes, plus about 1½ hour's rising

COOKING: about 40 minutes, plus cooling

15 g / ½ oz linseeds

15 g / ½ oz sesame seeds

15 g / ½ oz poppy seeds

About 225 g / 8 oz unbleached plain white bread flour, plus more for sprinkling and dusting

225 g / 8 oz wholemeal flour

1 heaped teaspoon ground sea salt

7.5 g / ¼ oz butter, diced, plus more for greasing

1 tablespoon honey

About 300 ml / ½ pint warm soya milk

15 g / ½ oz fresh yeast

Mix all the linseeds with three-quarters of the sesame and poppy seeds. Set aside. Sift the flours and salt into a large mixing bowl. Rub the butter into the flour with the fingertips. Blend in the reserved seed mix and make a well in the centre.

In another bowl, mix the honey into the milk and crumble the yeast into it. Mix well until dissolved. Pour the yeast mixture into the well in the flours and mix to a soft batter, beating until it leaves the sides of the bowl clean (you may have to add a little more white flour).

Shape into a round, put in a buttered bowl and turn to coat it in the butter. Cover with a tea towel and leave to rise until doubled in size, about 1 hour.

Knead into a long cylinder and cut this into about 8 pieces. Roll each into a sphere. Sprinkle the surface with the remaining poppy and sesame seeds and roll each sphere over them to cover the sides and top. Set well apart on a baking sheet and leave again to rise until doubled in size, about 30 minutes.

Preheat the oven to 230°C/450°F/Gas 8. Bake the rolls for about 40 minutes, until golden and sounding hollow when tapped on their bases. Allow to cool on wire racks.

CORN BREAD

P ★★★   E ★★   A ★

This traditional bread (see photograph, page 10) from the southern USA works well in both a sweet and savoury context. It is good spread with no-added-sugar jam or as an accompaniment to dishes such as Hoppin' John (see page 107). Corn is a source of potassium and the soya milk and caraway seeds provide phytoestrogens.

MAKES a 23-cm/9-in square loaf

PREPARATION: about 20 minutes

COOKING: 20–25 minutes

Olive oil or butter for greasing

85 g / 3 oz wholemeal flour

150 g / 5 oz fine yellow cornmeal

2½ teaspoons double-acting baking powder

¾ teaspoon salt

2 eggs

1–2 tablespoons honey

40 g / 1½ oz butter, melted

250 ml / 9 fl oz soya milk

2 teaspoons caraway seeds

Preheat the oven to 220°C/425°F/Gas 7 and grease a 23-cm/9-in square cake pan. Put it in the oven to heat.

Sift the flour, cornmeal, baking powder and salt into a large bowl and make a well in the centre. In another small bowl, beat the eggs, then beat into them the honey and melted butter, followed by the milk. Pour this into the well in the flours and combine quickly with a few stirs until a smooth batter. Stir in the caraway seeds.

Pour into the hot pan, smooth the top and return to the oven. Bake for 20–25 minutes, until golden and firm to the touch. Serve, cut into squares.

FOUR-SEED LOAF

P ★★★★   E ★★★★   A ★

Seeds are an excellent source of essential oils and phytoestrogens.

MAKES 1 large loaf
PREPARATION: about 30 minutes,
plus 2–2½ hours' rising
COOKING: 35–40 minutes, plus cooling

25 g/1 oz sesame seeds

25 g/1 oz linseeds

25 g/1 oz poppy seeds

25 g/1 oz sunflower seeds

15 g/½ oz fresh yeast

1 tablespoon honey

425 ml/15 fl oz lukewarm water

325 g/11½ oz unbleached white bread flour, plus more for sprinkling and dusting

325 g/11½ oz wholemeal bread flour

15 g/½ oz sea salt

1 tablespoon olive oil, plus more for greasing

Mix the seeds together in a bowl and set aside. Crumble the yeast into another small bowl and mix with the honey and 4 tablespoons of the lukewarm water until smooth.

Mix the flours and three-quarters of the mixed seeds together with the salt in a large mixing bowl. Make a well in the centre and tip in the yeast mixture, followed by the rest of the lukewarm water and the olive oil. Draw a little flour in from the edge until you have a smooth thick batter in the well. Sprinkle the surface of the batter with a little flour and leave for about 20 minutes, until the batter is spongy.

Gradually mix the remaining flour from the outside edges into the batter and work until it gathers into a ball, leaving the sides of the bowl clean. Turn out on to a lightly floured surface and knead for about 10 minutes, turning it as you do so, so it is stretched in different directions. Shape again into a smooth ball, put in an oiled bowl and turn to coat it with the oil. Cover with a damp tea towel and leave to rise in a draught-free place for about 1–1½ hour(s), or until doubled in size (it is perfectly risen when it doesn't spring back when pressed).

Using the knuckles, knock the dough back in the bowl, then turn out on the floured surface and shape it into a round or oval as you wish. Sprinkle the remaining seeds over the surface and roll the loaf in them to coat it, pressing the seeds in with your hands if necessary. Place on a baking sheet, cover with a damp tea towel and leave to rise again for about 1 hour, until doubled in size.

Preheat the oven to 220°C/425°F/Gas 7.

Uncover the loaf and cut a deep cross in the centre if round or diagonal slashes across the top if oval. Bake the loaf for 15 minutes, until lightly browned, then reduce the oven setting to 190°C/375°F/Gas 5 and bake for 20–25 minutes more, until the loaf sounds hollow when the base is tapped.

Allow to cool on a wire rack.

PHYTO BARS

P ★★★★   E ★★★★   A ★

These make good energy-giving snacks at any time of day, as well as delivering good quantities of phytoestrogens. They are perfect for carrying with you for whenever your blood sugar begins to drop. This recipe has a good level of plant hormones from all the seeds (the linseeds in particular) and, of course, essential fatty acids.

MAKES about 12
PREPARATION: about 15 minutes
COOKING: about 15 minutes, plus cooling

Olive oil and butter for greasing
450g/1lb honey
1 tablespoon lemon juice
85g/3oz sesame seeds, lightly toasted
85g/3oz sunflower seeds, lightly toasted
85g/3oz poppy seeds
85g/3oz linseeds

Lightly oil the insides of a large heavy-based pan and butter a Swiss roll tin.

Put the honey and lemon juice in the pan, mix well and bring to the boil (without any further stirring) over a moderate heat. Then, stirring constantly, boil to a temperature of 138°C/280°F to 'soft crack stage' (a little of the syrup dropped into iced water stretches into hard but elastic strands). Immediately take off the heat and stir in all the seeds, combining well, then quickly pour into the prepared Swiss roll tin and set aside.

After it has cooled for about 10 minutes, use a wetted knife to mark it into about 12 bars. When completely cool, cut or break the bars apart. Store in an airtight tin, interleaved with waxed paper to prevent sticking.

FRUITY HALVAH

P ★★★   E ★★★   A ★

These bars make a delicious, healthy snack as well as a dessert. They contain sesame seeds which are rich in calcium. Sesame seeds are also phytoestrogenic, as are the soya milk and cinnamon. Try to favour dried fruit that almost crystallises when dried, like dates and pineapple.

MAKES about 36 bars
PREPARATION: about 10 minutes, plus several hours' chilling
COOKING: about 30 minutes, plus cooling

250ml/9floz honey
1 litre/1¾ pints soya milk
200g/7oz butter
250g/9oz fine semolina
85g/3oz sesame seeds
Large pinch of ground cinnamon
100g/3½oz mixed dried fruit, finely chopped

Make a syrup by mixing the honey and the milk and bringing to the boil, stirring all the time, then boil for about 15 minutes.

In a large heavy pan, melt the butter over a low heat and add the semolina, seeds and cinnamon. Cook, stirring constantly, until the seeds brown lightly. Add the milk syrup and stir to mix. Cover and simmer for 5 minutes, until it develops the consistency of a thick paste. Allow to cool slightly.

Stir in the dried fruit and pour out over a baking sheet lined with rice paper. Use a wetted palette knife to spread it over the paper in a flat rectangle. Cover with another piece of rice paper and weight this down with a tray and some tins. Leave it in a cool place for a few hours or overnight.

Cut into long bars to serve.

OATCAKES

P ★ ★ ★   E ★   A ★

You can buy ready-made oatcakes from
supermarkets and health food shops but they do
not taste nearly as good as these. Oats are
phytoestrogenic and, with their facility for
lowering cholesterol, are also excellent for
the heart.

MAKES 24
PREPARATION: about 15 minutes
COOKING: about 30 minutes, plus cooling

Olive oil or butter for greasing
450 g/1lb medium oatmeal, plus more for dusting
1 teaspoon freshly ground sea salt
1 teaspoon bicarbonate of soda
115 g/4oz butter, melted
About 175 ml/6 fl oz hot water

Preheat the oven to 150°C/300°F/Gas 2 and lightly
grease 2 large baking sheets.

Mix the oatmeal, salt and bicarbonate of soda in a
mixing bowl. Stir in the melted butter and then
pour in just enough of the water to bind the
mixture to a firm dough.

On a surface dusted with more oatmeal, knead
the dough briefly to remove cracks, then divide it
into 6 pieces. Roll each of these out to a round
about 5mm/¼in thick and 20cm/8in across. Cut
each of these into quarters, brush off any loose
oatmeal and arrange on the prepared baking sheets.

Bake for about 30 minutes, until firm and crisp.
Allow to cool on wire racks.

SUGARLESS SPONGE

P ★ ★ ★   E ★   A ★

This is a lovely treat, which is not naughty but is
nice. Turn the sponge into a trifle using sugar-
free jam, fresh fruit and All Natural Custard
Powder (see page 44 for details), or simply split
and fill with sugar-free jam or lemon frosting
(see facing page). Alternatively, you can fill it
with tofu cream (see page 183), which is very
tasty and will boost its phytoestrogen content.

MAKES a 23-cm/9-in round sponge
PREPARATION: about 25 minutes
COOKING: 25–35 minutes, plus cooling

85 g/3oz slightly salted butter, plus more for the pan
125 g/4½oz flour, plus more for dusting
3 large eggs
6 tablespoons honey

Preheat the oven to 180°C/350°F/Gas 4. Butter the
insides of a 23-cm/9-in cake pan, then line it with
baking paper and butter that. Dust the insides of the
lined pan with flour and shake out any excess.

Warm the butter gently until just pourable but
not oiling; leave it to cool slightly. Sift the flour into
a bowl. In another bowl set over a pan of hot water,
whisk the eggs with the honey until the mixture is
thick and the whisk leaves a trail when lifted. Take it
off the heat.

Sift one-third of the flour into the egg mixture
and fold it in as lightly as possible. Repeat with two
more batches of flour. Fold a little of this batter into
the softened butter and then fold that back into
the batter.

Pour into the prepared pan and bake for 25–35
minutes, until the cake starts to shrink from the
edges of the pan.

Run a knife around the edge of the pan to loosen the sponge, turn it out and allow to cool on a wire rack before removing the lining papers.

Variations: you can give extra flavour – and phytoestrogens – to the basic sponge in lots of ways by adding to the batter: the grated zest of a lemon or orange, 2 teaspoons of ground cinnamon or 1 tablespoon of lightly toasted fennel seeds or caraway seeds.

CARROT AND OLIVE OIL CAKE

P ★★★★★   E ★★★   A ★★★★

With its high antioxidant content, carrot cake is marvellously good for combating free radicals and preventing premature ageing. The important antioxidant beta-carotene is not only present in the carrots, but also in the apples and orange juice. Carrots, in conjunction with the soya flour and tofu, produce the very high phytoestrogen levels in this cake. Essential fatty acids are supplied by the walnuts and the tahini from the lemon frosting.

MAKES a 20-cm/8-in cake
PREPARATION: about 40 minutes
COOKING: about 1 hour, plus cooling

150 ml/¼ pint olive oil, plus more for greasing
85 g/3 oz wholemeal flour
85 g/3 oz plain white flour
2 tablespoons soya flour
1 scant tablespoon baking powder
2 teaspoons ground cinnamon
½ teaspoon freshly ground sea salt
150 ml/¼ pint honey

3 eggs, lightly beaten
2 teaspoons vanilla extract
Grated zest of ½ orange
85 g/3 oz chopped walnuts, plus some unchopped walnut halves to decorate
175 g/6 oz carrots, finely grated
2 sweet dessert apples, grated

FOR THE LEMON FROSTING:
115 g/4 oz soft tofu
1 teaspoon tahini
4 tablespoons maple syrup, or to taste
3 tablespoons lemon juice

Preheat the oven to 180°C/350°F/Gas 4 and line a 20-cm/8-in cake pan with baking paper, then oil the paper.

Sift the flours, baking powder, cinnamon and salt into a large mixing bowl (tossing in the granules left in the sieve at the end).

In another large mixing bowl, mix the oil with the honey, eggs, vanilla and orange zest. Add to the flour mixture and blend in well. Fold in the nuts and grated carrots and apples.

Pour into the prepared pan and bake for about 1 hour, until a skewer inserted into the cake comes out clean.

Let cool in the cake pan for about 15 minutes, then turn out, remove the paper and allow to cool completely on a wire rack.

While it is cooling, make the lemon frosting: put all the ingredients in a blender or food processor and process until smooth. When the cake is cool, spread this frosting over the top and decorate with some walnut halves. Leave at room temperature for an hour to let the frosting firm up a little.

Variation: you can make twice as much frosting, split the cake and fill it with a layer of frosting prior to topping.

DATE BAKLAVA

P ★   E ★★   A ★

This lovely dessert (see photograph, page 24) contains three different kinds of nuts, which are good sources of essential fatty acids. Dates are high in magnesium ('nature's tranquilliser') as well as potassium, which is so useful in preventing water retention.

MAKES about 60 pieces
PREPARATION: about 35 minutes
COOKING: 45–60 minutes, plus cooling

Olive oil or butter for greasing

85 g/3 oz walnut halves

85 g/3 oz blanched almonds, lightly toasted in a dry frying pan

85 g/3 oz pistachios, shelled and chopped

15 sheets of filo pastry

115 g/4 oz butter, melted

225 g/8 oz dates, coarsely chopped

1 tablespoon honey

½ teaspoon ground cinnamon

FOR THE SYRUP:

450 ml/¾ pint date syrup

½ teaspoon ground cinnamon

Small pinch of ground cloves

Juice and zest of ½ small lemon

2 tablespoons orange flower water

Preheat the oven to 160°C/325°F/Gas 3 and generously grease the insides of a deep 20-cm/8-in square cake tin.

Put the walnuts, almonds and pistachios in a food processor and pulse until reduced to the consistency of small breadcrumbs.

Cut the sheets of filo roughly to the size of the cake tin, keeping them under a damp tea towel when not in use or they will dry out and become brittle. Arrange 3 sheets in the bottom of the tin, painting each with melted butter and trimming as necessary.

Mix together the ground nuts, dates, honey and cinnamon. Sprinkle one-quarter of this mixture over the filo base. Continue with layers of buttered filo sheets and nut mixture until all are used up, finishing with a final 3 layers of buttered filo. Brush the top of this thoroughly with butter and sprinkle with 1 tablespoon of water.

Bake for 45 minutes, then increase the heat to 220°C/425°F/Gas 7 and cook for a further 10–15 minutes, until puffed up and lightly golden.

During this last phase of cooking, mix together all the syrup ingredients in a pan and bring to a simmer. Simmer gently for about 10 minutes. As soon as the baklava comes out of the oven, pour this syrup mixture over it and allow to cool in the tin.

To serve, slice at angles to make 2-cm/1-in long lozenge shapes.

Basics

MISO BROTH

P ★ ★ ★ ★ ★   E ★   A ★ ★

This miso broth is a wonderful store of phytoestrogens, not only from the miso (soya bean paste) but from the parsley and garlic too. Miso itself is so versatile that you can use it with many casseroles and soups: all you have to do is mix a tablespoon of miso into a small bowl with either hot water or liquid from the dish you are cooking and then add it back into the dish. Once you have added miso to a dish you should not bring it to the boil, otherwise its beneficial enzymes are destroyed.

MAKES about 850 ml/1½ pints
PREPARATION: 10 minutes
COOKING: 30 minutes minimum, preferably 1 hour

1 small onion or 2–3 shallots, chopped
1 garlic clove, chopped
Handful of parsley stalks (without the leaves)
1 tablespoon miso

Put the onion, garlic and parsley in a pan with 1 litre/1¾ pints of water and bring to the boil, then lower the heat, cover and simmer for about 30 minutes to an hour. After this time, pour a little broth into a small bowl, and stir in the miso to make a paste. Then add to the pan of broth, stirring well to mix in.

Variations: if you use the broth for an Oriental dish, add a few slices of root ginger with the onion and garlic. Miso broth is also tasty with added seaweed kombu, which brings extra nutrients.

COURT-BOUILLON

P ★ ★   E ★   A ★ ★

This is the aromatic liquid you should use for the poaching of fish, as it both adds flavour and minimises any flavour lost from the fish to the liquid. After use, you can keep it for the next time you cook fish (keep it in the fridge and/or boil it up from time to time to keep it sweet), This way it develops in strength of flavour.

The court-bouillon will deliver a number of phytoestrogens from the carrots and celery. Celery is an especially beneficial vegetable: it contains good amounts of potassium which can prevent water retention, and it also has anti-inflammatory properties.

MAKES about 3 litres/5¼ pints
PREPARATION: about 10 minutes
COOKING: 15 minutes, plus cooling

1 onion, chopped
2 celery stalks, chopped
2 carrots, chopped
150 ml/¼ pint dry white wine
1 bay leaf
Juice of ½ lemon
1 teaspoon black peppercorns
Freshly ground sea salt

Put all the ingredients in a large pan with 2.5 litres/4½ pints of water. Bring to the boil and boil for about 10 minutes, skimming, then leave to cool slightly.

Season to taste with salt and then strain over the fish to be cooked.

VEGETABLE STOCK

P ★★   E ★   A ★★★★

This stock keeps well, covered, in the refrigerator for up to a week or frozen for up to 1 month. If you are going to reduce it down for a sauce, etc, don't add any salt.

You can use stronger-flavoured vegetables like fennel, cabbage and leek to add body to the stock, but be careful not to use too much of any one such vegetable or it may overpower the other flavours.

The stock contains an excellent variety of antioxidants from the vegetables and also phytoestrogens from the broccoli, carrots and the celery.

MAKES about 3 litres/5¼ pints
PREPARATION: 15 minutes
COOKING: about 1¼ hours

1.8 kg/4 lb mixed vegetables, preferably including carrots, onions, broccoli, French beans, celery stalks and tomatoes, coarsely chopped
Large handful of parsley stalks, chopped
1 garlic clove, halved (optional)
1 small red chilli (optional)
1 bay leaf
1 teaspoon black peppercorns
150 ml/¼ pint dry white wine
Freshly ground sea salt

Put all the ingredients except the salt in a large pot, add 4 litres/7 pints of cold water and bring to the boil.

Reduce the heat to a gentle simmer and cook gently, uncovered, for about 1 hour.

Strain through a fine sieve, discarding the solids, and season to taste with salt.

FISH/SEAFOOD STOCK

P ★★   E ★   A ★★

If you buy your fish from a good old-fashioned fishmonger they are usually only too happy to supply you with the trimmings from your fish – and any others that happen to be lying around. Try to avoid trimmings from oily fish like mackerel – even salmon – as these give too strong a flavour. The fennel, carrots and parsley in the stock all offer phytoestrogens, and the carrots are rich in the important antioxidant, beta-carotene.

MAKES about 850 ml/1½ pints
PREPARATION: about 15 minutes
COOKING: 30 minutes

1 kg/2¼ lb fish or seafood trimmings, such as bones, heads (gills removed), tails, shells, etc
1 onion, chopped
2 fennel stalks, chopped
2 carrots, chopped
Large handful of parsley stalks, chopped
150 ml/¼ pint dry white wine
Juice of ½ lemon
1 teaspoon black peppercorns
Freshly ground sea salt

Thoroughly rinse the fish trimmings and put them in a large pot with the remaining ingredients, except salt, and 1 litre/1¾ pints of cold water. Bring to the boil slowly and skim carefully.

Lower the heat and simmer gently for 30 minutes (no more or the fish bones will start to give off bitterness), skimming from time to time.

Strain through a fine sieve, discarding the solids, and season to taste with salt.

BASIC TOMATO SAUCE

P ★★★   E ★   A ★★★★

This keeps well in a covered container in the refrigerator for up to a week. Packed full of antioxidants from the lycopene in the tomatoes, the sauce also contains phytoestrogens from the miso, garlic and parsley.

MAKES about 900 g/2 lb
PREPARATION: about 15 minutes
COOKING: about 35 minutes

2 tablespoons olive oil

1 large onion, chopped

1 garlic clove, finely chopped

100 ml/3½ fl oz red wine (optional)

400 g/14 oz tinned chopped plum tomatoes

3 tablespoons tomato paste

1 tablespoon parsley, chopped

1–2 teaspoons miso dissolved in 300 ml/½ pint boiling water

Freshly ground sea salt and black pepper

Heat the oil in a heavy-based pan and sauté the onion in it gently until just translucent, then add the garlic, and sauté for about 1 minute more. Add the wine (if using) and boil rapidly to reduce it to a sticky liquid.

Stir in the tomatoes with their liquid, the tomato paste, parsley and miso broth. Mix well, season and simmer for about 30 minutes, until it has a thick sauce-like consistency.

TOMATO KETCHUP

P ★   E ★   A ★★★★

Tomato ketchup is a staple of nearly every household's cupboard, but the shop-bought version is unfortunately full of sugar. This version is so much better for you, and so much better tasting. It will keep for one to two weeks in the refrigerator, covered. It is packed with antioxidants (from the tomatoes and red wine in particular) and other excellent ingredients including ginger, which is good for circulation.

MAKES about 450 g/1 lb
PREPARATION: about 20 minutes
COOKING: about 30 minutes

Two 400 g/14 oz tins of chopped plum tomatoes

1 onion, finely chopped

1 garlic clove, very finely chopped

3 tablespoons cider vinegar

3 tablespoons red wine (optional)

3 tablespoons tomato paste

3 tablespoons honey

1 teaspoon finely grated fresh ginger or ½ teaspoon ground dried ginger

Good pinch of ground allspice

Good pinch of ground cloves

Good pinch of ground mace

Good pinch of celery salt

Freshly ground sea salt and black pepper

Purée the tomatoes with the onion and garlic in a food processor until smooth (you may need to do this in batches). Tip into a heavy-based pan and stir in the remaining ingredients with seasoning to taste. Bring to a simmer and cook gently for 30 minutes, or until nice and thick, stirring from time to time.

BLENDER MAYONNAISE

P ★   E ★★★★   A ★

This is a very unusual mayonnaise in that it is made with linseed oil, which contains valuable essential fatty acids. As mayonnaise is made from raw eggs and doesn't get cooked, you do have to be careful about possible salmonella levels. Make it from very fresh eggs bought from a reliable supplier, keep it (and dishes made using it) in the fridge and don't keep it (them) for more than a day or two. To be really safe, it's really not advisable to serve raw egg to young children, pregnant women or invalids.

MAKES about 300 ml/½ pint
PREPARATION: about 5 minutes

125 ml/4½ fl oz olive oil
125 ml/4½ fl oz linseed oil
1 large egg
Pinch of dry mustard powder
Freshly ground sea salt and black pepper
1 tablespoon cider vinegar or lemon juice
1 tablespoon boiling water

Try to ensure that all the ingredients are at the same room temperature before you begin. In a jug, mix the oils together.

Put the egg and mustard powder in the (ideally small inner) bowl of the food processor with seasoning to taste. Process until foaming, then add the cider vinegar or lemon juice and pulse to mix.

With the machine running, dribble in the mixed oils, almost drop by drop to begin with and then in a slow steady stream, pouring faster as the mayonnaise starts to thicken. Mix in the boiling water at the end to help make the mayonnaise more stable.

Variation: basic mayonnaise can be flavoured in a myriad of ways to suit different food: try adding 2–3 garlic cloves with the egg for a garlic mayonnaise that is wonderful with prawns or crudités; stir in some chopped parsley, chives and chervil at the end for a herb mayonnaise that goes with most fish and egg dishes; whizz in a bunch of watercress to make the most unforgettable dressing for boiled potatoes. (Also see Rémoulade Dressing, page 130.)

SOYA MAYONNAISE

P ★★★★   E ★★★   A ★

While not strictly a mayonnaise, this makes an excellent creamy dressing and is also rich in phytoestrogens, with its tofu and linseed oil content. Garlic is believed to have cancer-inhibiting properties.

MAKES about 150 ml/¼ pint
PREPARATION: about 5 minutes

150 g/5 oz soft tofu
55 ml/2 fl oz olive oil
55 ml/2 fl oz linseed oil
1 tablespoon soy sauce
2 garlic cloves, crushed
1 teaspoon Tabasco sauce
1 tablespoon lemon juice
Freshly ground sea salt and black pepper

Put all the ingredients in a blender or food processor and process until smooth, seasoning to taste.

BASIC VINAIGRETTE

P ★   E ★★★★★   A ★★

The linseed oil of this vinaigrette makes any salad deliver a good punch of essential oils. Use wine vinegar (white or red), balsamic vinegar or lemon juice according to what best suits the salad ingredients. For other phyto-packed dressings, see the Crushed Nut Vinaigrette on page 86, the Parsley Vinaigrette on page 94 and the Lemon Vinaigrette on page 144.

MAKES about 90 ml/3 fl oz
(enough for a side salad for 4)
PREPARATION: under 5 minutes

3 tablespoons olive oil
2 tablespoons linseed oil
1 tablespoon wine vinegar or balsamic vinegar, or lemon juice
Freshly ground sea salt and black pepper

Either beat all the ingredients together in a bowl using a fork or shake in a screwtop jar to emulsify. When adding the seasoning to taste, add only just enough salt so that the dressing no longer tastes oily.

SESAME TOFU DRESSING

P ★★★★   E ★★★   A ★

This creamy, phyto-packed dressing works well on most salads and lightly cooked vegetables. It is also rich in essential fatty acids. If you cannot get hold of white miso from health food shops, add some soy sauce.

The Austrian Bean Salad gives another interesting tofu dressing (see page 130).

MAKES about 250 ml/9 fl oz
PREPARATION: about 10 minutes

115 g/4 oz soft tofu
2 tablespoons sesame oil
1 tablespoon linseed oil
2½ tablespoons cider vinegar
2 teaspoons white miso or soy sauce
1 garlic clove, crushed
1 tablespoon mirin (Japanese rice wine)
1 tablespoon sesame seeds, lightly toasted

Put all the ingredients except the sesame seeds in a blender or food processor and process until smooth. Stir in the sesame seeds.

TOFU DIP FOR RAW VEGETABLES

P ★★★★   E ★★★★   A ★★★★

SERVES 4
PREPARATION: about 5 minutes

1 tablespoon sesame oil
1 teaspoon linseed oil
Freshly ground sea salt
½ teaspoon grated root ginger
225 g/8 oz soft tofu

Put all the ingredients in a blender or food processor and blend until smooth, adding just enough water, a little at a time, to get a good dipping consistency.

Variation: you can add a tablespoon or two of tahini for even more flavour and goodness.

PESTO SAUCE

P ★   E ★★★★   A ★

Pesto is an extremely useful thing to have in the fridge (it keeps better than mayonnaise) as it makes such an excellent tasty dressing for many vegetable dishes and can also serve as the easiest of pasta sauces. I think you get the best results by far using a good old-fashioned mortar and pestle, but you can simply whizz everything but the cheese in a blender and then stir in the cheese at the end.

The pesto sauce delivers an excellent selection of essential oils from the linseed oil and the pine nuts.

MAKES about 400 g/14 oz (12 good dollops)
PREPARATION: about 15 minutes

55 g/2 oz basil
25 g/1 oz pine nuts
2 garlic cloves
Freshly ground sea salt and black pepper
115 g/4 oz Parmesan cheese, freshly grated
6 tablespoons linseed oil
6 tablespoons olive oil

Using a mortar and pestle, pound the basil, pine nuts, garlic and a pinch of salt to a paste.

Mix in the cheese well, then beat in the oils, a little at a time. Adjust the seasoning with salt and, if you like although it is not strictly necessary, a little pepper.

Variations: these days pestos crop up made from all sorts of things; most commonly the basil is replaced with either parsley, coriander or anchovy.

HERB BUTTERS

P ★★★★   E ★★★   A ★★

These butters are wonderfully handy things to have in the fridge. A slice of dill or parsley butter makes the easiest and most appropriate dressing for grilled fish, and chive, mint or basil butter are great on grilled or boiled vegetables. You can even mix herbs, using, say, the classic *fines herbes* mix of parsley, chervil, chives and tarragon. Try this and other herb butters as an instant omelette filling or pasta sauce. Finely chopped garlic, chilli and root ginger can also work well given this treatment.

To boost the nutrition content of a simple herb butter, as you are mashing the herbs into the butter also mix in some linseed oil.

MAKES about 150 g/5 oz (10 pats)
PREPARATION: about 5 minutes, plus chilling

Handful of herb leaves (see above), finely chopped
Freshly ground sea salt and black pepper
115 g/4 oz softened unsalted butter

In a small bowl and using a fork, mash the herb(s) with seasoning to taste into the butter. Turn out on a sheet of greaseproof paper and roll into a cylinder. Chill until firm.

To use, cut off 15 g/½ oz slices as required.

RHUBARB RELISH

P ★★★　　E ★　　A ★★★

This relish goes particularly well with oily fish like mackerel or herring, or any spicy dish. Rhubarb is a source of phytoestrogens, the ginger is good for circulation and there are antioxidants in the orange juice and zest. Never cook rhubarb in an aluminium pan because the acidic nature of the vegetable leeches toxic aluminium into the food itself. Those suffering from arthritis should avoid rhubarb because of its oxalic acid content.

MAKES about 1.5 kg/3¼ lb
PREPARATION: about 15 minutes
COOKING: 1–2 hours

1 kg/2¼ lb rhubarb, cut into short pieces
225 g/8 oz dates, chopped
3 large onions, chopped
Juice and grated zest of 2 large oranges
5-cm/2-in piece of fresh root ginger, finely grated
225 g/8 oz raisins
1 tablespoon mustard seeds
1 cinnamon stick
350 ml/12 fl oz honey
500 ml/18 fl oz cider vinegar
Freshly ground sea salt and black pepper

Put all the ingredients in a large non-reactive pan with seasoning to taste, bring to the boil and simmer gently until thick (1–2 hours). Remove the cinnamon stick and adjust the seasoning if necessary.

Pour into warmed sterilised glass preserving jars (with glass lids) and seal. It will keep well for months and actually improves in flavour after a week or so.

PEANUT SAUCE

P ★★★★　　E ★★　　A ★★

This sauce is rich in nutritional goodies. The soya milk and garlic contain high amounts of phytoestrogens, the onions have a positive influence on bone health and the garlic is an anti-cancer ingredient. Use the sauce within a couple of days, and store it in the refrigerator.

MAKES about 450 ml/¾ pint
PREPARATION: about 30 minutes
COOKING: about 20 minutes

1 large red onion, coarsely chopped
3 garlic cloves
1–2 fresh red chillies, deseeded (optional)
175 g/6 oz skinned raw peanuts
2 tablespoons olive oil
1 tablespoon soy sauce
2 tablespoons tamarind paste, dissolved in 2 tablespoons water
150 ml/¼ pint soya milk
2 teaspoons honey
Freshly ground sea salt

Blend the onion, garlic and chilli (if using) in a blender or food processor until they form a paste.

Gently dry-roast the peanuts in a pan, stirring to avoid burning. Allow to cool. When they are cool, crush them in a food processor until finely ground.

Heat the oil in a wok. Add the onion paste and fry, stirring constantly, for 1 minute. Add the ground peanuts and stir until combined. Add the soy sauce, tamarind, soya milk and honey.

Gently cook until all the flavours are combined and a thickish sauce has formed (add a little water if necessary), about 15 minutes. Add salt to taste.

PEANUT BUTTER

P ★★   E ★★★★   A ★

It is best to keep this nutty spread in the refrigerator and use within a couple of days: you won't find this hard, as it is so tempting. It is full of essential oils, from the linseed oil.

MAKES about 250 g/9 oz
PREPARATION: about 10 minutes

225 g/8 oz skinned raw peanuts
4 tablespoons linseed oil
Freshly ground sea salt

Gently dry-roast the peanuts in a pan; do not burn. Allow to cool. In a blender or food processor, whizz the nuts and oil together to a paste (coarse or smooth as you prefer). Season to taste with salt.

MOCHA TOFU CREAM

P ★★★★   E ★★★   A ★★

This is a delicious coffee-flavoured 'cream' but without the usual heavy calories and saturated fat. It is rich in plant oestrogens from the tofu and essential oils from the almond butter. The raisins contain a good amount of potassium, which helps with water retention.

SERVES 2
PREPARATION: about 10 minutes
COOKING: 25 minutes

85 g/3 oz raisins
225 g/8 oz silken tofu
3 tablespoons almond butter
1 tablespoon instant grain coffee granules
(eg Caro Extra)
Pinch of freshly ground sea salt

Put the raisins in a pan with water to cover. Bring to a simmer and cook gently for 20 minutes. Drain the raisins and blend until smooth.

Squeeze as much water from the tofu as you can. In a blender or food processor, process the tofu, the raisin purée, the almond butter and the coffee granules until really smooth.

TOFU CREAM

P ★★★★   E ★   A ★

This makes an excellent substitute for dairy cream and can be used as a topping for a fruit salad or on any desserts where you would normally use cream.

SERVES 4
PREPARATION: about 5 minutes

225 g/8 oz soft tofu
½ teaspoon vanilla extract
100 ml/3½ fl oz maple syrup
1 tablespoon sunflower oil
1 teaspoon linseed oil

Combine all ingredients in a blender until smooth.

References

Introduction

1 V Beral et al, 'Breast cancer and HRT: collaborative reanalysis of data from 51 epidemiological studies of 52,705 women with breast cancer and 108,411 women without breast cancer', *The Lancet* (1997), 350, 9084

Understanding the role of oestrogen

1 V Beral et al, 'Breast cancer and HRT: collaborative reanalysis of data from 51 epidemiological studies of 52,705 women with breast cancer and 108,411 women without breast cancer, *The Lancet* (1997), 350, 9084

What you need to eat at the menopause

1 S Barnes et al, 'Rationale for the use of genistein-containing soy matrices in chemoprevention trials for breast and prostate cancer', *Journal of Cellular Biochemistry Supplement* (1995), 22, 181–187

2 H Aldercreutz et al, *The Lancet* (1992), 339, 1233

3 A Murkies et al, 'Dietary flour supplementation decreases postmenopausal hot flushes: effect of soy and wheat', *Maturitas-Journal of the Climacteric and Postmenopause* (1995), 21, 189–195

4 P Albertazzi et al, 'The effect of dietary soy-supplementation on hot flushes', *Obstetrics and Gynaecology* (1998), 91, 1

5 G Wilcox et al, 'Oestrogenic effects of plant foods in postmenopausal women', *British Medical Journal* (1990), 301, 905–906

6 Source: US National Cancer Institute

7 J Ziegler, 'Soybeans show promise in cancer prevention', *Journal of the National Cancer Institute* (1994), 86, 1666-1667

8 H Aldercreutz et al, 'Dietary phytoestrogens and cancer: *in vitro* and *in vivo* studies', *Journal of Steroid Biochemistry and Molecular Biology* (1992), 3–8, 41, 331–337

9 SP Verma, 'Curcumin and genistein, plant natural products, show synergistic inhibitory effects on the growth of human breast cancer MCF-7 cells', *Biophysical Research Communications* (1997), 233, 3, 692, 696

10 C Gennari, 'Introduction to the Symposium', *Bone Mineral* (1992), 19, S1-S2 and JB Anderson et al, 'The effects of phytoestrogens on bone', *Nutrition Research* (1997), 17, 10, 1617–1632

11 FS Dalias et al, 'Dietary soy supplementation increases vaginal cytology maturation index and bone mineral content in postmenopausal women', Second International Symposium on the Role of Soy in Preventing and Treating Chronic Disease (1996, Brussels, Belgium)

12 HM Linkswiler et al, 'Protein-induced hypercalciuria', *Federation Proceedings* (1981), 40, 2429-2433 and BJ Abelow et al, 'Cross-cultural association between dietary animal protein and hip fracture: a hypothesis', *Calcified Tissue International* (1992), 50, 14–18

13 Source: M Messina et al, *The Simple Soybean and Your Health* (1994, Avery Publishing, New York)

14 NA Breslau et al, 'Relationship of animal protein-rich diet to kidney stone formation and

calcium metabolism', *Journal of Clinical Endocrincology and Metabolism* (1988), 66, 140–146

15 MJ Stampfer et al, *New England Journal of Medicine* (1985), 313, 1044–1049

16 J Anderson et al, 'Meta-analysis of the effects of soy protein intake on serum lipids (1995), *New England Journal of Medicine,* 333, 5, 276–282

17 DE Pratt et al, 'Source of antioxidant activity of soybeans and soy products', *Journal of Food Science* (1979), 44, 1720–2

18 G Dhom, 'Epidemiology of hormone-dependent tumours' in *Endocrine-Dependent Tumours,* KD Voigt and C Knabbe eds (1991, Raven Press, New York)

19 MS Morton et al, 'Lignans and isoflavonoids in plasma and prostatic fluid in men: samples from Portugal, Hong Kong and the United Kingdom', *The Prostate* (1997), 32, 122–128

20 SB Bittiner et al, 'A double-blind, randomised, placebo-controlled trial of fish oil in psoriasis', *The Lancet* (1988), I, 378–380

21 J Kremer et al, 'Effects of manipulation of dietary fatty acids on clinical manifestation of rheumatoid arthritis', *The Lancet* (1985), I, 184-187 and F McCrae et al, 'Diet and arthritis', *Practitioner* (1986), 230, 359–361

22 H Aldercreutz, 'Lignans and phytoestrogens: possible preventive role in cancer' in P Rozen ed. *Frontiers of Gastrointestinal Research,* Vol 14, (1988, Karger, Basel, Switzerland) 165–76

23 LB Taubman, 'Theories of ageing', *Resident and Staff Physician* (1986), 32, 31–37

24 AA Bertilli et al, 'Antiplatelet activity of cis-resveratrol', *Drugs under Experimental and Clinical Research* (1996), 22, 2, 61–63

25 J Levy et al, 'Carotene and antioxidant vitamins in the prevention of oral cancer', *New York Academy of Sciences* (1992), 260–269

26 E Middleton and G Drzewieki, 'Naturally occurring flavonoids and human basophil histamine release', *International Archives of Allergy and Applied Immunology* (1985), 77, 155–157

27 M Gabor, 'Pharmacologic effects of flavonoids on blood vessels', *Angiologica* (1972), 9, 355–374

28 JD Cohen and HW Rubin, 'Functional menorrhagia: treatment with bioflavonoids and vitamin C', *Current Therapeutic Research* (1960), 2, 539–542

29 J Monboisse et al, 'Oxygen: free radicals as mediators of collagen breakage', *Agents Actions* (1984), 15, 49–50

30 GE Abraham, *Journal of Nutritional Medicine* (1991), 2, 165–178

31 AK Bordia et al, 'Effect of garlic oil on patient with CHD', *Artherosclerosis* (1977), 28, 155–159

32 I Yamamoto et al, 'Anti-tumour effects of seaweed', *Japanese Journal of Experimental Medicine* (1974), 44, 543–546

33 N Iritani and S Nagi, 'Effects of spinach and wakame on cholesterol turnover in the rat', *Atherosclerois* (1972), 15, 87–92

What you don't need to eat or drink at the menopause

1 TL Holbrook and E Barrett-Conner, *British Medical Journal* (1993), 1056–1058

2 A Komori et al, 'Anticarcinogenic activity of green tea polyphenols', *Japanese Journal of Clinical Oncology* (1993), 23, 3, 186–190

Index

Shopper's guide

Here is a list (in alphabetical order) of various brands that I know to be of good quality:

Food brands

Aspell   01728 860510
Cider vinegar

Biona   020 8395 9749
Linseeds

Cauldron Foods   01275 818448
Organic tofu

Doves Farms   01488 684880
Organic wholemeal flour

Just Wholefoods   01285 651910
Natural custard powder

Life and Health   01322 337711
Worcestershire sauce, horseradish sauce, sunflower dressing

Meridian Foods   01490 413151
Range of natural products

Provamel   020 8577 2727
Organic soya milk (plain)

St Dalfour   01727 834215
Sugar-free jams

Vintage Roots   01189 761999
Range of organic wines by mail order

Whole Earth   020 7229 7545
Range of natural products

Yeo Valley   01278 652243
Natural organic yoghurt

The following are wholefood stores, some of which are able to send products by mail order:

Stores

Nutri Centre   020 7436 5122
Range of natural products; also mail order

Olivers   020 8948 3990
Natural wholefood store; also mail order

Freshlands   020 8395 9749
Natural wholefood store; also mail order

Planet Organic   020 7727 2227
Natural wholefood store

Wild Oats   020 7229 1063/0468
Natural wholefood store

These supplements containing phytoestrogens are ideal for when you are away from home (see page 43):

Supplements for travelling

Novagen Red Clover   08705 329244 *(mail order)*
                     0845 603 1021 *(helpline)*
Red clover supplement (40mg of isoflavones)

PhytoSoy   08705 329244 *(mail order)*
Herb tea containing phytoestrogens

Staying in touch

If you have any health problems and are interested in a more natural approach to treating them, or would like to find out what supplements and tests are available to you, please feel free to contact me on the number below. I will send you information on how you can help yourself.

Workshops, cassettes and videos
I occasionally give workshops and talks around the country and have produced cassettes and videos from some of these. Please get in touch if you would like to find out more about future workshops and/or the recordings, and you will be sent an information pack.

Consultations
If you feel the need to see or talk to someone personally, I am available for private consultations at the following clinics:
The Hale Clinic, Regent's Park, London
TLC, St John's Wood, London

For appointments and enquiries:
Tel: 01892 750511 Fax: 01892 750533
www.marilynglenville.com
email health@marilynglenville.com
Dr Marilyn Glenville
Nevill Estate
Danegate
Eridge Green
Tunbridge Wells TN3 9JA

If you would like to hear more advice from Dr Marilyn Glenville on any of the following subjects:

Natural alternatives to dieting – how to lose weight naturally

Natural alternatives to HRT – how to stay healthy through the menopause and prevent osteoporosis

Natural alternatives to infertility – how to increase your chances of conceiving and preventing miscarriages

Then call: 0906 7010030 and select the information required.

ACKNOWLEDGEMENTS

This book could not have been written without the help and support of friends and colleagues.

I would particularly like to thank Lewis Esson for his invaluable contribution to the recipes and for his ability to incorporate unusual ingredients to make such delicious dishes. My thanks also to Candida Hall, my editor at Kyle Cathie, who worked so quickly and with such patience. I would also like to express my appreciation to Kyle Cathie and her superb team for all their support and encouragement. Thanks also to Teresa Hale of the Hale Clinic and Mr Mehta of the Nutri Centre.

While I have been busy writing, my practice manager Linda McVan and all the staff at the Natural Health Practice – Brenda, Bea, Lous and Trisha – have been working in the background, making it possible for me to complete this book.

My love goes to my family, Kriss, Matthew, Leonard and Chantell for all their support and continued interest in whatever I am working on.

Photographs shown outside the recipe section are as follows: